BURNOUT & BEYOND

DON EASTON

Copyright © 2022 Donald T Easton

All rights reserved. Except for the quotation of small passages for the purposes of criticism or review, no part of this publication may be reproduced, stored in a retrieval system or transmitted in any form or by any means, electronic, mechanical, photocopying, recording, scanning or otherwise, without the permission in writing of the author.

Although the author and publisher have made every effort to ensure that the information in this book was correct at press time, the author and publisher do not assume and hereby disclaim any liability to any party for any loss, damage, or disruption caused by errors or omissions, whether such errors or omissions result from negligence, accident, or any other cause.

Scripture quotations marked NLT are taken from the Holy Bible, New Living Translation, copyright ©1996, 2004, 2015 by Tyndale House Foundation. Used by permission of Tyndale House Publishers, Carol Stream, Illinois 60188. All rights reserved.

Scripture quotations marked TPT are from The Passion Translation®. Copyright © 2017, 2018, 2020 by Passion & Fire Ministries, Inc. Used by permission. All rights reserved. ThePassionTranslation.com.

Scripture quotations marked NIV are taken from the Holy Bible, New International Version®, NIV®. Copyright © 1973, 1978, 1984, 2011 by Biblica, Inc.™ Used by permission of Zondervan. All rights reserved worldwide. www.zondervan.com The "NIV" and "New International Version" are trademarks registered in the United States Patent and Trademark Office by Biblica, Inc.™

Scripture quotations marked MSG are taken from THE MESSAGE, copyright © 1993, 2002, 2018 by Eugene H. Peterson. Used by permission of NavPress, represented by Tyndale House Publishers. All rights reserved.

Kindle Edition, License Notes

This eBook is licensed for your personal enjoyment only. This eBook may not be re-sold or given away to other people. If you would like to share this book with another person, please purchase an additional copy for each recipient. If you're reading this book and did not purchase it, or it was not purchased for your use only, then please return to your favourite eBook retailer and purchase your own copy. Thank you for respecting the hard work of this author.

ISBN: 9798836368999

Imprint: Independently published
Cover design: Josh Easton

To Adrienne, my wonderful wife,

thank you for loving me. Your love and support helped me heal and gives me strength. You held on to me.

Thank you for being true to your word...

> *For better, for worse,*
>
> *For richer, for poorer,*
>
> *In sickness and in health,*
>
> *To love and to cherish,*
>
> *As long as we both shall live.*

To our children and their spouses: Sarah & Matthew, Josh & Katrina and Kate & Ashley who love me and prayed with me; Thank you.

CONTENTS

Foreword iv

Why a Book on Burnout? ii

How Does Burnout Begin? 1

The Fog of Burnout 25

Recovery: Rest & Replenishment 56

Creating Gauges 81

Preventing Burnout 104

Life After Burnout 130

Thank You Letters 140

ACKNOWLEDGMENTS

The gratitude I have for the people who have helped me through burnout is overwhelming. So many people lent their support in so many different ways, and without them, I would be in a very different, much darker place right now. It is truly through the love and help of those around me, that I made it through. It takes a village to raise a child, and it also takes a community to improve a person's health.

I have heard many stories, and seen examples firsthand, of organisations severing ties with their leaders who were entering burnout. This didn't happen to me, thanks to my extraordinary community. I am so thankful for the care I received when I was vulnerable and for all of those who made it safe when I was in a dangerous place.

I am grateful for my Christian heritage— my parents, Keith & Edith Easton, took me to church before I could walk.

Thank you to my wife Adrienne, my children, their spouses and children. Their love and support was my light in the dark.

Thank you, Ps Phil & Chris Pringle and C3 Church for the opportunity to minister and serve as Senior Minister for the last thirty years, including ten years as National Operations Manager serving the

Australian National Directors. C3 Church Robina and the Australian C3 Church Executive gave me space to get well and prayed for my recovery. I so appreciate my supportive friends in our global family.

Thank you, Ps Gordon Moore for your friendship and the strength of your leadership in our journey.

Thank you to my life-changing mentor, Dr Keith Farmer, who helped develop my self-awareness, build a practice of self-reflection, and empower self-moderation in my life. Your mentoring helped me reinvent myself.

Thanks to Dr Chris Adams, Azusa Pacific University, who led the Health of a Christian leader class I attended and presented his scientific research in well-being. Chris has become a friend who helped me through this journey. Also, thanks to Dr Arch Hart for his significant work and writings in this field, and his three daughters; Dr Sharon Hart May, author of *Safe Haven Marriage*, Dr Sylvia Hart Frejd, author of *Digital Wellness* and Dr Catherine Hart Weber author of *Emotional Wellness*, who also presented in this class. Their expertise added clarity and articulation to my experiences.

Thanks to Dr Bob Logan, my professional coach since 2018, whose encouragement, support and guidance has really helped me to develop these ideas and transform them into a coherent guide for others. I greatly appreciate our friendship and transformative coaching.

Thank you to Cecelia Meserve for bringing order and readability to my words, research and learning with your wonderful word craft.

Thank you to my wife, Adrienne, for your editing prowess from my first theological paper to editing this book.

Foreword

It was my first time going to church camp as a High School student. I had the time of my life and made some important spiritual decisions at that camp, including solidifying a call to vocational ministry. I also learned that one of the highlights of camp was to sneak out of our cabin at night and run around the campground. It was a bit of a game to get chased by the youth pastors and counsellors. So, not wanting to be left out of the fun, I snuck out of the cabin with some buddies. None of us had been to the campground before. We were sprinting across the campground in the dark, feeling invincible. What we did not know was that there were waist-high posts about every five feet, lining the main drive through the camp...and in between the posts was a thin, metal wire. One of my friends and I were out in front of the group running full speed when our legs hit the wire. We were thrown back several feet in the air by the collision and laid there simultaneously in shock, laughing at the comedic value of the moment and also in pain. Our friends who were behind us were laughing as well and told us that we looked like we ran into some kind of invisible forcefield. Slightly injured, we recovered and kept running. As we ran back to the cabin, we also did not see a black clothesline in the dark. Four of us simultaneously caught the clothesline at face level and were laid out on our backs. I now had injured legs and a fat lip because I did not know about the hidden dangers and did not bother to ask anyone who had snuck out of the cabin before—I kept on going anyway. You have the blessing of learning from someone who knows the hidden hazards of ministry as you read this book.

Through research and clinical work, I have heard countless pastors say something like, "I was blindsided…It hit me out of nowhere…I didn't see it coming." There is something about the insidious nature and onset of burnout that is such that it hides from the ministry leader. The truth is that burnout can accumulate outside our awareness, becoming suddenly apparent when it hits a threshold of severity. Burnout can even happen when things are going well in ministry. This all-too-common phenomenon is why I am so excited about this book.

"Pastors don't get into difficulty because they forget that they are pastors, but because they forget that they are persons". This is perhaps my favourite quote from my dear friend and mentor, the late Dr Archibald Hart. He was one of the first psychologists to systematically research clergy stress and burnout and work with pastors to prevent severe cases. After co-teaching with him late in his career, I was privileged to have inherited his course in the Doctor of Ministry program at Fuller Theological Seminary. The course, "The Personal Life of the Leader", is the longest-running course in the history of

Fuller's DMin program. Alums often return multiple times to repeat the course as they encounter stress throughout their ministry careers. Dr Hart was decades ahead of his time, as more current research only underscores and validates his intuition starting in the 1970s and 1980s. The insights from this trajectory of scholarship are included in the pages of this helpful book.

It was through teaching Dr Hart's course that I met Dr Don Easton. As Don and I spent some time together both in class and outside of class, I learned about his compelling story that he shares in this wonderful resource. I was struck by the depth of Don's authenticity, which research demonstrates is a key dimension of flourishing in ministry. He has truly lived the journey through burnout and beyond and is allowing God to redeem the painful chapters of his own story by becoming equipped to lead and support other pastors. Don has done the difficult, personal work of recovery and has created a sustainable rhythm to avoid repeating burnout in his own life. He has also done the hard work of research and professional growth to become a leading voice in his culture and times. Don has years of rich experience in leading other clergy into healthier, sustainable rhythms. Like all great pastors, Don has synthesized complex scholarship, life and ministry leadership experience, and Biblical and theological principles to create a contextualized, practical resource accessible to all. This resource is especially timely given the impact of ministry stress during the global pandemic and whatever the new normal looks like for clergy. Don artfully dispels some of the common myths of ministry burnout and provides invaluable insights and practical advice that can keep pastors from being blindsided and impaired. May our Lord Jesus Christ restore the joy of your salvation and the joy of ministry as you implement the recommended practices in the pages that follow.

Sincerely,

Rev. Christopher J. Adams, PhD.

Chris Adams, PhD, grew up in a music ministry family in the Nashville area. He is a third-generation pastor's kid and an ordained minister. He served in full-time music ministry for several years after college, then as an associate pastor at a large church for 5 years during and after seminary. He also provided pastoral care to missionary families while completing doctoral work at Fuller Theological Seminary. Adams recently completed 8 years as the associate campus pastor for pastoral care at Azusa Pacific University, and is serving as executive director of the Centre for Vocational Ministry, which focuses on cultivating resilience in ministry leaders and students through research and formational resources. He also teaches ministry leadership and pastoral care/counselling courses in Azusa Pacific Seminary. Adams is a consultant to a number of denominations and seminaries in the areas of clergy candidate assessment, clergy health, and pastoral leadership formation, and is participating as a consultant, researcher, and writer with the Duke Clergy Health Initiative, Profiles in Ministry Project for the Association of Theological Schools, and the Flourishing In Ministry project at the University of Notre Dame. Adams is also a frequent lecturer at seminaries, retreats, and conferences.

ENDORSEMENTS

"Don has written with honesty, courage and humility, addressing the issue of emotional depletion and burnout at a time when pastors are being affected in unprecedented numbers.

It has been a privilege to support Don as a mentor for about 8 years, and to rejoice at his recaptured health, vitality and passion to help other pastors.

The gauges he presents are particularly helpful for anyone seeking to recover from emotional depletion.

I highly recommend this excellent book."

Dr. Keith Farmer
Mentor, Principal Emeritus, Australian College of Ministries. Doctor of Ministry, Fuller Theological Seminary.

"Don Easton's book, Burnout and Beyond, is personal, timely and refreshing… much needed for the men and women in ministry today. He provides ways to identify the signs of burnout, strategies for coping and building resilience, and hope for coming out stronger on the other side.

I'd recommend that every Christian leader, whether currently on the path to burnout or not, read this book. It will help them maintain health, replenish their energy when needed, and reduce the stigma around burnout so they and others are attuned to the signs and can help guide others on the path to healing and replenishment."

Dr. Robert E. Logan
Author of *An Undivided Heart* and *The Leadership Difference*

"Comprehensive and easy-to-read, Easton's 'Burnout & Beyond' weaves together personal story with a wealth of factual information and practical steps. The great strengths of the book lie in Don's honesty and realism and his consistent grounding in Christian faith. Every phase of dealing with burnout is addressed here: prevention, assessment, immediate and medium-term responses, recovery and rebuilding. Particularly helpful is his section on creating gauges to track signs relevant to the onset and recovery from burnout. 'Burnout and Beyond' will be tremendously useful for all Christian leaders and for their spouses and friends. Even if you don't think you require this right now, I highly recommend it for vital awareness of an issue that urgently needs to be better understood."

Dr Rick Lewis
Author of Mentoring Matters, Chair of Australian Christian Mentoring Network, Founder of Anamcara Consulting

"My friend Don has faithfully served as senior minister with C3 Global for over 30 years and sharing from his own journey brings a book that will help so many. Burnout is a significant problem today. Don's book helps us understand the problem and gives pathways to recover and thrive again. He gives us good news that we can get through whatever we face."

Ps Dr Phil Pringle AOM
Global President C3 Church

"Burnout and meltdowns seem to be the lot of producers; they simply don't know when or even how to stop, much less listen. I'm not sure Don's sage advice (and it is certainly worth listening to) will stop the process, but what he has written will definitely help you navigate your way out, and, in his parlance, find a richer and more enduring future – something he is now enjoying.

Don has disarmingly invited us the inner workings and processing of a very painful time in his life. His honesty is the first step to healing, his willingness to listen the second, and his self-awareness the key to maintaining a healthy, less driven, and fulfilling lifestyle. He shows that there is light on the other side of darkness.

The text is full of wise advice, helpful steps, and excellent resources. Don writes to all situations, having read and studied widely, and not that of his profession only. As you read, I'm sure you'll be confronted, challenged and thereby changed – hopefully.

I unreservedly recommend Dr Don Easton's story to you."

Simon McIntyre
C3 Church Global Team; Americas

"The pressures and challenges of leadership contribute directly to the increasing stories of adrenaline exhaustion and burnout. In this excellent book, Don shares his own story with great courage and vulnerability, offering us much needed wisdom and many practical insights for staying healthy over the long haul. Highly recommended."

Dr Mark Conner
Speaker, Author, Trainer, Coach

"It has been a pleasure working with Don over the past few years. Following his studies at Fuller, he brought back considerable expertise in mentoring people to avoid burnout and stay true to mission. We have been so impressed by his expertise that a wide selection of our senior staff consult regularly with him as part of keeping their professional, spiritual and family life on track. This has now continued for a number of years and is a testimony to his theoretical knowledge, practical knowledge and expertise. All professionals in ministry will benefit from engaging with Don and his work."

Rees Davis
Executive Principal, King's Christian College

"When you are going through any kind of crisis the best person to look to is one who has been there done that and survived! Don Easton's book Burnout and Beyond draws from the wellspring of his own personal journey through burnout to recovery. Don humbly describes the subtle and gradual nature of his decline into the valley, the challenges and struggles back to a place of healing and restoration, and the deep lessons learned along the way.

This book outlines clearly the deep causes of burnout and its symptoms. It also gives real tools for evaluating your emotional health and wellbeing and outlines some very sound and practical steps for a holistic approach to recovery. Best of all it gives hope that burnout is not "the end destination but can be a path to a better, stronger you." If you have experienced the pain of burnout, feel like you are heading towards it, or simply want to avoid it altogether, Don's book will prove invaluable."

Ps Wayne Peat
Coordinator C3 Pacific Pastor's Support

"In all my years of ministry I'm not sure I can recall a time when I sensed that so many leaders/ministers were feeling weary, under pressure and certainly a lot less motivated than they would hope to be. So, to say that Don's book is timely is an understatement.

When I reconnected with Don a few years ago I was struck by the deep peace, humility and calmness in his life. Yes, he's walked the path of burnout, but he has also slowly and intentionally walked the path of healing too.

I encourage leaders to read this book and grasp the invaluable wisdom and practical insight–but most importantly–I encourage leaders to read this inspirational story of truth, hope, recovery–and above all the grace of our wonderful God."

Rev Dr Graham Humphris
Chairperson Generate Presbytery UCASA

"In Burnout & Beyond Don Easton shares vulnerably about his personal journey of burnout and recovery. This book is filled with practical, research-based solutions to help guide you to a place of better health. It is a must-read for anyone living with high demands."

John Finkelde
Founder, Grow a Healthy Church

"In his book Burnout and Beyond, Don Easton provides us with an insightful and practical guide for identifying, dealing with and discovering wholeness in his journey with burnout. He combines this with some very helpful professional guidelines as well."

I highly recommend this book to anyone experiencing burnout and also to leaders, family, professionals and associates in order to gain a greater understanding of burnout and the way forward to healing and wholeness."

Dr Gordon Moore
Emeritus Senior Minister, C3 Lighthouse Bridgeman Downs

"Don has always been one of those 'real deal' kind of people. He lives what he says and articulates with great clarity what he means.

This book reflects this throughout, as he reveals his own journey through burnout, his observations from both inside and outside of burnout, and the inclusion of professional narrative to help either someone approaching or in a burnout, or someone close supporting someone going through it.

This would be one of the clearest and most succinct helps you could get your hands on!"

Steve & Lizby Warren
Founder: https://beautifulminds.global/
Senior Pastors - C3 Imagine, Regional Director - C3 Europe

INTRODUCTION

Why a Book on Burnout?

February 2014 was the first time my General Practitioner told me I was burnt out. After weeks of insomnia, anxiety and heart palpitations, I finally went to see him, convinced that something was wrong with me. I assumed it was a physical illness, not an emotional one. I have been a church planter and a senior minister at C3 Church Robina for decades. The job comes with many stressors—managing others, writing sermons, handling conflict—but all were stressors I felt I was handling. I was shocked when my GP said I was suffering burnout and needed to take time off to recover. My psychologist diagnosed High Stress, Moderate Anxiety and Mild Depression, and on doctor's orders, I ceased work in April 2014. My claim with WorkCover was approved. After six months off work, dedicating myself to rest and replenishment, I started back at twelve hours a week with a gradual increase over the next twelve months.

Burnout is a common term for a condition whereby a person

experiences physical and emotional repercussions after doing a difficult job for a long time. Studies show that thirty-three per cent of adults will experience burnout at some point in their lives, sometimes with debilitating symptoms. I have seen it firsthand: pastors who were once vibrant and vital in their ministry finding themselves exhausted and challenged to muster the motivation and energy for ministry work. Like a cat stalking a mouse, it feels as if a shadow lurks behind you never allowing you to rest completely. Some never fully recover.

The journey through burnout is a long, often dark, road. It was one of the most challenging times in my life, and I could never have gotten through it without the help of others. On the other side of the experience, I want to share what I have learned in the hope that I can help others facing this sort of depletion. I have spent years recording and reflecting on what led me to burnout and how I was able to come out stronger. I eventually developed a series of gauges to track a person's emotional health and prevent burnout.

This book's fundamental limitation, and perhaps its strength, is that it is written from life experiences. It is not a clinical perspective. I'm not a professional psychologist or a psychiatrist. I do not hold a formal education in those areas, but I do have formal education in ministry and a wealth of experience. I have spent most of my life helping others in crisis and mentoring and coaching people. I began Verve Lead[1]; a not-for-profit registered charity focusing on well-being mentor training, providing tools and consulting. The goal is to lift Christian leaders' buoyancy and resilience and enhance our communities' well-being, sustainability, and safety. Much of my work focuses on preventing and aiding others through burnout in a well-being mentoring capacity.

In addition, I have spent nearly a decade studying and researching burnout and have built relationships with some of today's leading psychologists and coaches specialising in emotional well-being.

While I have learned and grown through this period of my life and have much to share, note that my reflections are not a replacement for professional help and that self-diagnosis is often inaccurate. This book should serve as a guide to support others if they find themselves on this path, *in addition* to the help they seek professionally. I would also like to point out that there are many different faces of burnout, and my stories won't speak to everyone. My experience is within the ministry world, and much of my research has revolved around burnout in the church. However, I believe that anyone heading towards burnout can benefit from rest and reflection, understanding what it is and how to

---

1 Vervelead.com

prevent reoccurrence. This book is for anyone approaching burnout, experiencing burnout, recovering from burnout. It's also for the people around them to help support and love them through this difficult time.

I have several goals in writing this book:

- To help identify burnout.
- To assist in reducing burnout.
- To help the process of healing.
- To build self-awareness around things that deplete and replenish, thereby preventing further episodes.
- To reduce the stigma of burnout.

I know what it is like to feel broken, and I know what it is like to be in the process of mending. These days, am I a hundred per cent? No. Some things that I was strong at, I am just not good at anymore, yet I have grown stronger in other areas. After this experience, I don't want to be the same. The thought of dealing with the same stress, fears and limitations sends a shiver down my spine. But counter to that, a feeling of gratitude rises in me. I smile, knowing that I am different from the man I used to be. If anyone reading this feels like there is no light at the end of the tunnel, there is. Things will get better, and you will come out the other side, stronger but different. And that's a good thing.

4 He always comes alongside us to comfort us in every suffering so that we can come alongside those who are in any painful trial. We can bring them this same comfort that God has poured out upon us.

— 2 Corinthians 1:4 (The Passion Translation)

CHAPTER ONE

How Does Burnout Begin?

My Background

Many would say that my life and ministry were successful. As a young man of twenty-one years, I left my employment as a clerk at a motor parts manufacturer to take a position in a country church, reaching out to the town's youth. I believed that God, whom I had given my life to, would fill me with His Spirit and work through me. I believed that He who called me would provide for me because the position was voluntary with some limited payment for pizza and petrol (the two essentials needed for a youth minister). I learned to have faith in God for his provision, praying for supply and resources. Miraculously, God provided all I needed: a new car battery, clothes, holidays, money, friendships and Adrienne, whom I would marry the following year.

I was inspired to enrol in a ministry training college while working as a youth minister. I had failed at school, both year 11 and 12. My spelling and grammar were abysmal. My theology professor handed back my first paper with the words in red at the bottom of the first page, "*I will not bother to mark this rubbish until you correct your grammar and spelling.*" I persevered, believing that He who calls me is faithful. Adrienne, a junior primary teacher, taught me to spell and write correctly. Graduating with a Bachelor of Theology and Graduate Diploma of Ministry, I was ordained into the Uniting Church Ministry as a minister of the word and sacrament. I commenced parish ministry in Yorke Peninsula, South Australia, looking after five congregations.

During this time, the voice of the Spirit spoke to me again, telling me I should get my doctorate. After laughing at God for a few months and giving him a list of more suitable candidates, I commenced my doctorate at the Fuller Theological Seminary Doctor of Ministry program. Partway through, I was invited to plant a church in the new city called Robina in South-East Queensland. Adrienne and I accepted and, under supervision by Fuller during the ministry project phase of the Doctor of Ministry, planted Robina Uniting Church.

We were four years into growing the new congregation and involved in purchasing a multi-million-dollar site for a new complex when it became clear that the church's leadership and my leadership had different philosophies. Believing that God still called us to this area, we began again.

We connected with C3 Church (then called Christian City Church), finding them the glove that fitted. This time we were not resourced by a denomination but again relied on God's faithfulness for provision. It was a challenging time emotionally as I felt rejected and cut off from my mother church. My new church family was gracious and gently ministered to and bandaged my wounds. The church struggled in that first year, but by God's grace, it grew as people came to faith and others joined us to build. God's provision was such that I continued to be paid the same wage.

Sometime later, our movement leaders asked us to become the State Directors overseeing the South Australian churches. Later, we became the Queensland State Directors, which included mentoring a young couple who eventually became State Directors after us. This role was followed by a National role as Operations Manager, working alongside the National Director. I worked in this role two days a week for ten years.

At this time, we purchased 2.2 hectares (6 acres) of land, and after some initial difficulties, we were finally able to move the church on site. Our church grew to four congregations after the move: Youth on Friday evening, two Sunday morning and one Sunday evening. The church we planted grew to nearly 500 people (at least 80 per cent of

USA churches are under 200 in attendance).

Our church team was humming, impacting locally, nationally, and even internationally by helping to establish churches in Papua New Guinea. The team was one of high capacity, talented, dedicated people. But as Carl George says, "Even extraordinary talent and extra-mile dedication cannot prevent eventual burnout[2]."

Many would consider my personal life to be successful as well. Adrienne and I were married in 1979. We worked hard to create an honest and intimate relationship. Our three married children all loved God and were involved in church life. We enjoyed a close relationship with them and their spouses. Six months before seeing early signs of burnout, Adrienne and I moved to a property we wanted to develop by building a new home on a subdivided lot. We were expecting our first grandchild. Things were good, and there was a lot to be excited about.

Calling my life and work 'successful' does not sit comfortably with me now. Now, instead of 'successful', I prefer to say I was granted the ability to see that God loves me and has a purpose for my life. I set about following that purpose. Great fulfilment and joy came in helping others know Christ as I had come to know him. However, I

---

2 George, Carl F.. How to Break Growth Barriers: Revise Your Role, Release Your People, and Capture Overlooked Opportunities for Your Church (p. 194). Baker Publishing Group. Kindle Edition.

viewed success in the outcomes measured by the world. I placed a high value on statistics: the size of our congregation, the money we brought in, the amount of growth—important things for any leader in ministry, but, looking back, I had lost some of my initial values. I wanted success by numbers more than I wanted a nurturing and thriving community. I wanted so badly to achieve that I neglected my emotional health, injuring myself and others around me.

Cracks begin to appear

After about five years in the new church building, the cracks appeared, not in the facility but in the team. Gordon Moore acknowledges in his book *Going to the Next Level*[3] that churches heading towards a congregation of 500 is a big step. "Many pastors experience burnout at this stage as they try to blend the demands of a large church with family commitments and the increasing number of opportunities to influence and impact beyond their own church that comes with proven fruitfulness and experience." A larger church places larger demands on the leaders. This is what we experienced.

Within a month of each other, two key assistants went on burnout leave. Even though I helped them through the challenges, and I had

---

3 Moore, Gordon. *Going to the Next Level* (Ark House Press, 2015)

seen and helped colleagues and their churches, I see now that I had very little understanding of burnout. We tried as best we could to care for our key assistants and set about replacing them with four people. As the key driver of the bus, I took on more of the weight, thinking it was my responsibility to fill the gap by working both more and harder. I endeavoured to take on the role of training the new team.

We were running at an unsustainable pace with the high level of personal exertion required. Looking back, as hindsight is usually 20/20, it's easy to see that we were in big trouble—I could not see it at the time. We began to have a decline in attendance. As the church shrank, so did the number of services. We went to three, to two, to one. Good people who had key roles in the church, and had given so much to build the church, began to leave.

I felt increasingly rejected and let down. I spoke of disloyalty and justified it by saying, "Jesus is pruning his church." I was blind to a growing problem in myself. In this blindness and pain, I shrank back from conflict and avoided moments when I needed to give corrections. My team was lacking spiritual sustenance and not feeling empowered. As they tried to address the problem, they spoke of the symptoms. Although it was not their intention, I felt attacked: good people were just trying to find words for the difficulties they saw. One common comment was, "I am not getting anything from [your] sermons." Unable to see that something was wrong in me, I presumed it was because they were drinking from other ponds, listening to the best of the best online, getting sustenance from somewhere else. These were people who had experienced God in our church through my preaching. Many had met Jesus there, but not anymore. They simply hungered to meet him again.

My blindness grew along with my emotional difficulty. I took criticism personally more and more. I am grieved for the pain I caused. Emotions boiled and words were spoken that should not have been spoken. I wonder now how the church survived this. I can only acknowledge that it's His church, and He is the one who holds the parts together.

Eventually, burnout caught up with me.

Is it the weak who burn out? No!

I'm embarrassed to acknowledge this, but I thought those prone to burnout were weak. For too long, mental and emotional illnesses have been seen as flaws rather than something that can happen to anyone. Writing this now makes my prior attitude seem so foolish. It's like thinking that a child with lymphoma did something wrong to catch the sickness or saying that a person with the flu is at fault for feeling awful. What did they do wrong to cause it to happen? Yes, there may be contributing factors—lifestyle contributes to health—but so much is out of our control. Essentially, our role is to do what we can to see the sick healed when possible.

Burnout has a considerable stigma attached, partly because it is still not well understood. I was so wrong with my attitude towards burnout, and it took my own experience to show me the truth. Part of my quest has become demystifying burnout to reduce blame and guilt. Opposite to my prior attitude, it's often the *strong* who are more likely to burn out: the people who want to make a difference, those with courage and tenacity, those who are willing to push to see a change. Caretakers of all kinds are the most susceptible because they are more prone to pushing themselves too hard. It has been heartening to see more and more strong leaders openly talking about their burnout experiences.

Many great people have walked this journey. It is not limited to a professional group. Almost anyone in any job can burn out. While it is partly the duty of an employer to care for his workers by limiting negative factors within the workplace, even the most thoughtful employer can find burnout in his employees. There is a deeper, underlying problem in how our society lives life. We tend to care primarily about where we will end up and how fast we can get there, rather than focusing on the present journey. Yet, the journey often shapes our destination: the struggles and pleasures encountered to reach a goal give that goal more value.

I love riding motorbikes. I've enjoyed riding several, from fast racing bikes to heavy cruisers. As a seventeen-year-old, it was all about going fast on an RD 350 two-stroke Yamaha. Once, while accelerating, redlining through the six gears, the throttle stuck on approach to a T-intersection. I hit the kill switch, locking up the back brake and came to a stop just before the corner. I dismounted the bike, shaking with adrenaline, feeling very thankful I had not crashed. These days, I still enjoy the occasional ride on a fast bike, but I much prefer to just go for a ride. The destination is not the consideration, or who gets there first and fastest. Instead, it's all about the ride—enjoying the time with fellow riders and the feeling of life that floods my soul as I cruise. My experience with burnout made me realise I was living my life like my seventeen-year-old self—fast and dangerous. It was neither sustainable nor enjoyable. Now I try to focus on the journey as it happens. I try not to rush, just to take things as they come.

As you read on, you will understand what causes burnout: too much stress over a long time. 21st century understanding and measurement of success compound this stress. High-performance, high-capacity people willingly and consistently put themselves under pressure to see their cause come to reality. This book will help you build a more sustainable life and aid you to employ healthy practices that will allow you to flourish. You may need to pull back from your responsibilities, but with help, you can continue.

So, please don't beat yourself up if you are heading towards burnout, are burnt out, or have suffered from burnout in the past. Don't consider yourself weak because of this difficulty or put yourself down. Read on and hopefully understand why people become burnout in the first place. Keep travelling through this challenging season until you find a place of healing. You will get better and come out with a more vital understanding of yourself.

Adrenaline and Stress Birth Burnout

Adrenaline is designed to be our friend. The body releases it in times of danger to give us strength for fight or flight; a surge of energy that can save our lives in a time of emergency. But it is meant to be released sparingly and not remain at a constantly high level. Arch Hart outlines the effect of a high level of adrenaline. "The high level of adrenaline sparked by stress reduces our ability to rest. It cuts down on our apparent need for sleep and creates poor eating habits. All this can lead to increased usage of drugs, alcohol, cigarettes, and other damaging substances. These, in turn, can take their toll by causing further illnesses and damage in and of themselves. So too much stress can set in motion a long chain of destructive side effects."[4]

When did I start living on adrenaline? My production of a high level of adrenaline is linked to my personality. I like to be in control, and losing that control leads to adrenaline and stress. My leadership role means I have a lot of responsibilities in a wide variety of areas: I can often be working with complicated schedules, rushing from event to event. I am often mediating conflict and disagreements between employees. I need to understand the big picture of my work while also dealing with the small, everyday details required to get the job done. There are times in leadership when there is an increasing gap between desired outcome and current reality. The less control I feel in my work, the more stressed I become.

Arch Hart, in his exceptionally helpful book *Adrenaline and Stress,* says, "recent research shows that when a person is caught up in a situation about which he or she feels helpless with no control over the outcome,

---

[4] Hart, Archibald. Adrenaline and Stress: The Exciting New Breakthrough That Helps You Overcome Stress Damage . Thomas Nelson. Kindle Edition. Location 273 or 3840

cholesterol as well as adrenaline levels increase significantly."⁵

My own life is evidence of Hart's research—my solution to my stress was to do more and go harder, thereby drawing more and more on adrenaline to fuel me. The constant diet of adrenaline became an addictive high. I continued to do my work and live my life, but I had no idea what a mess I was making for myself in the future.

Signs of this began to show physically and emotionally. In *Adrenaline and Stress,* Hart says, "It's the same with muscle tension. It goes up when stress demands it but doesn't necessarily come down when the stress is gone. The result is usually chronic headaches, backaches, and nervous tics."⁶ For me, the early signs were increased muscle tension in the back, neck and quads, tight hamstrings, and a feeling of emotional numbness. Remedial massage became a necessary relief. I was lucky— for some people, stress shows in heart attacks and strokes.

I pushed on until the adrenaline ran out. We had just completed a National Conference for which I had a significant role in organising. Usually, I would be on a high after such an event, feeling satisfied that I

---

5 Hart, Archibald. Adrenaline and Stress: The Exciting New Breakthrough That Helps You Overcome Stress Damage (Kindle Locations 335-337). Thomas Nelson. Kindle Edition.

6 Hart, Archibald. Adrenaline and Stress: The Exciting New Breakthrough That Helps You Overcome Stress Damage (Kindle Locations 335-337). Thomas Nelson. Kindle Edition.

could add value. This time was very different. When I returned home, I felt numb. I lost my decision-making ability. When Adrienne asked, I couldn't even choose where we would go for dinner. I kept saying, "I just want to lie down."

Hart says, "The problem with our dependence on high levels of adrenaline is that we have to pay the piper for this abuse later on. What it amounts to is accelerated "wear and tear" on our cardiovascular systems, creating burnout—much like a high-performance car that has been allowed to overheat."[7]

Now, it is easy to see how foolish I was to push myself to a breaking point. But I could not see the danger in which I had placed myself and others. The sickness made me blind and irresponsible. Thankfully, my story does not end here.

A Note for Those Approaching Burnout

Are you approaching burnout? Maybe your GP or a mentor has said that they see you stretched too thin or running on adrenaline. My most significant piece of advice is to listen to professionals and those who care about you. Take their advice. Be encouraged that healing will

---

[7] Hart, Archibald. Adrenaline and Stress: The Exciting New Breakthrough That Helps You Overcome Stress Damage (Kindle Locations 335-337). Thomas Nelson. Kindle Edition

come. Strength will return. Resilience will grow. This difficulty can be a gift that can help you reinvent yourself.

If you have enough clarity of mind, read on, understand what is happening, and how to make some positive changes. The good news is that it is much easier to recover if you catch yourself before experiencing severe burnout. You can avoid the pain and cost by taking the time *now* to rest and replenish. Hopefully, you will be back on your feet soon, more aware of your boundaries.

A Note for The Burnt Out

If you have arrived at burnout, you are likely experiencing a feeling of emptiness. It is unfamiliar and scary. You will think that you just don't have the energy you used to have. I want to say that you are not going to stay here. You can get better.

One of the very common side-effects during this time is a feeling of failure for the inability to be there for others. You compare yourself with who you were before; you see all the things you used to do for the people you care about, and you feel you are letting them down because you are not doing these things anymore. Often, the burnt-out withdraw, tempers get shorter, apathy grows. No matter what it looks like, you have changed, and it will affect those closest to you. These things can cause a strong sense of shame and self-blame to grow. However, this is not the time for self-condemnation. It is not the time for beating yourself up. Blaming yourself will not help you get better.

Burnout is an injury that comes from high exertion and high activity. Your emotions have become depleted as you have worked and pushed yourself hard. You have been making a difference. You have been in the fight and have come out alive. I salute the champion you are! Hold your head high, knowing that what you feel is because you have worked hard and given so much. But now it's time to give to yourself. It's time for your rest and healing. The people who love you will understand.

If you have been given this book because of severe burnout, you may not have the energy or focus on reading further. Follow the advice of the professionals assisting you. Rest. As healing and restoration begin, come back to this book. That's the time to pick it up again. You will go beyond burnout. Burnout is not the end destination but can be a path to a better, stronger and more whole you.

A Note to Those Who Know Someone in Burnout

Is your emotional tank full? Are you securely and comfortably attached to the people in your world? Do you have overall high satisfaction with life and your accomplishments? If this is you, you are probably not suffering from burnout. However, if someone in your life is burnt-out, know that it can (and likely will) affect you at some point. This book will be valuable to you.

Burnout is an epidemic in our society, easily seen by the alarming increase in the prescription of antidepressant medication (although burnout is not the only reason people are prescribed antidepressant medication). According to the Australian Bureau of Statistics, 1.7 million people (7.8% of the Australian population) had at least one PBS subsidised prescription for antidepressant medications filled in 2011. Therefore, you will probably encounter someone who will go through this debilitating sickness, if not in your family or friends, then in one of your work colleagues. They will be feeling alone and scared, and you can be a safe place for them. So, read on as I give some actions for what to do if you think someone is approaching burnout:

- Learn the signs of burnout.
- Listen to the person. Set a safe space and encourage them to talk about what they are experiencing and how they are feeling.
- Don't diagnose them or let them self-diagnose. Seek a professional's opinion.
- If you see some signs, don't isolate or criticise them, even if you are frustrated. Know that their behaviour is a symptom of

burnout.

- Don't take on their burnout alone. Seek help for them and yourself so you can both get through this period of struggle.

I am so grateful to Adrienne and my family for their love and support during my burnout journey. Their steadfast, unconditional love provided the atmosphere needed for healing.

My Spouse is Going Through Burnout: by Adrienne Easton

Being the spouse of a person going through burnout has unique difficulties. Indeed, how do we even approach the topic with them if we suspect that they are nearing burnout? This is not easy if your spouse is running on adrenaline, is highly motivated in work, and becomes defensive when the topic is brought up.

I had an episode of depression and burnout back in 2009/10. While I knew that something was wrong, and Don saw it too, I was stubbornly determined to ignore the symptoms. It seemed there was too much life at stake to let go and rest. Finally, Don arranged a meeting with our overseer, a close female pastor and friend. It was this third-party perspective that permitted me to finally see that I was unwell and in need of counselling, medical intervention, and time away from responsibilities to recover. I did buck at taking time out. I believed I should keep working, perhaps subconsciously thinking that my church wouldn't cope without me. It was during a session with my counsellor that God gave me a beautiful picture of how my resting and subsequent recovery ministered to Him as well as me. I thank God for those who spoke into my life during this time.

Often, we neglect to listen well to our spouse when we are not coping, perhaps because we try to ignore our situation, hoping that we'll improve without intervention, or maybe because we don't want to burden our spouse further. Of course, though, this only exacerbates our situation as we internalise our disappointments and frustrations. And then finally, the result is worse for both our spouse and us. So, if you suspect that your spouse is approaching burnout, seek counsel from a person you trust and who has a voice of authority in your life.

Pray. Always pray. God is on your side. Pray for your spouse to have self-awareness and to be willing to listen to you. Pray for soft, loving words as you initiate conversations about symptoms you have noticed.

We may fight with feelings of rejection by the one person we thought would always be present and listening in conversation, always buoyant, approachable and engaging. We may think, "Who is this person? This is not the person I married! This one drinks too much, falls asleep in front of the TV, then keeps me awake because he tosses and turns and snores; he gets defensive when I talk about difficulties, is irritable with me and the kids, is easily critical, withdraws to his phone…" Ah, yes, sometimes it feels like we are flying solo, and our wingman has dropped off the plane.

All these are symptoms of Don's burnout that I saw before he accepted the fact. So, what helped me to still love him through the journey and for our marriage to come out strong? Perhaps the greatest factor is the knowledge that during my period of depression and burnout, he did all he could to make space for me to do so and get the help I needed. He drove me on the long trips to see my counsellor and let me sob all the long drive home. He understood that depression was not something I could recover from in my strength. He prayed for me continually. So, of course, when Don burnt out, I was there for him with the understanding that he would recover and that I would do all I could to assist in that journey. Besides, when we were married in 1979, we vowed to "love and care, in sickness and in health", and I am a woman of my word.

Secondly, knowing that burnout is a sickness helped me cope with the feelings of rejection that initially surfaced through Don's behaviour. He was not intentionally hurting me by disregarding me. He was so depleted that he was incapable of giving out as he had done before.

Also, all the small steps along the way to Don's recovery were signs that one day he would be his strong, vibrant self again. God reminded me of the man with whom I had spent thirty-three years of marriage—the characteristics I loved about him, how he was committed to our marriage and of the special moments we had shared. That kept me hopeful and resolute. He would be restored. If your spouse or someone close to you is on the recovery journey, I encourage you to ask God for a picture and a scripture to cling to as you support, love, and do all you can to see them healed.

Finding Comfort During Burnout

The severity of burnout is measured in the amount of stress, anxiety and depression a person experiences. These symptoms can form a pit with slippery and deep walls, leaving you feeling trapped. Often the methods you've used in the past to replenish yourself no longer work. Sometimes, the pit becomes so deep that you may have no desire to get out, let alone to see the possibility of doing so. It feels hopeless. I remember feeling adrift in a fog, floating on an ocean, and not being able to see where land was, not knowing if I would or could make it back to the shore.

Then like a bell in the fog on the sea, I heard a still voice say, "*The Lord is my shepherd. I shall not want.*" With those words came a deep knowing in my heart that it was going to be okay despite my sickness. Then as the days went by, I thought, "What does okay mean? Will I get better? Will I live a life of significance?"

Several months passed and I was not better. I wondered again if I would make it. Some people close to me assured me that I would get well; their voice didn't inject me with instant strength to swim strongly to the shore but rather gave me the confidence to keep resting in the current.

I found Psalm 23 another reassuring voice; allowing me to trust the process and trust in the Lord:

¹ The LORD is my shepherd;
I have all that I need.
² He lets me rest in green meadows;
he leads me beside peaceful streams.
³ He renews my strength.
He guides me along right paths,
bringing honour to his name.
⁴ Even when I walk
through the darkest valley,
I will not be afraid,
for you are close beside me.
Your rod and your staff
protect and comfort me.
⁵ You prepare a feast for me
in the presence of my enemies.
You honour me by anointing my head with oil.
My cup overflows with blessings.
⁶ Surely your goodness and unfailing love will pursue me
all the days of my life,
and I will live in the house of the LORD Forever.
(NLT)

Therefore, listen for God's voice; what is he saying to you? Even though you walk through the darkest valley, don't be afraid, for the Lord is close beside you. Listen also to trusted friends. Listen to my voice in this book. You will get through this.

Reflection Questions for Chapter One:

1) What is my attitude towards burnout?
2) Who in my life has experienced burnout?
3) What have been my stressors in the past?
4) What are the main stressors in my life right now?
5) What steps do I need to take if I am burning out or burnout?

CHAPTER 2

The Fog of Burnout

What is Burnout, anyway?

When my medical doctor diagnosed me with burnout, I did not understand what it meant. I could hardly understand what was going on inside of me, much less find the words to explain it. When I realised that I was indeed burnt out, and once I finally accepted that, I wanted to know what I was facing. Over that year, through the help of my doctor, psychiatrist and well-being coach, I learned a lot about this condition. I also did some research of my own.

I have come to understand that knowing the components of burnout, recognising it and understanding how it affects people are necessary for providing a safe path for recovery.

In this chapter, I will share my experience, outline some key contributing factors, and expand on the main components of burnout.

Signs of Trouble

Do you know the fable of the boiling frog? A frog is dropped in a pot of lukewarm water; slowly, the heat is turned up degree by degree, so gradually that the frog doesn't realise he is being boiled. I was the frog, unaware of the rising heat, just swimming. It took a long time to recognise that something was wrong. In hindsight, it's elementary to see I was in an unhealthy place, but it can be difficult to see yourself clearly in the middle of burnout.

The first thing I was able to register was feeling very flat. In December of 2013, I felt exhausted all the time and apathetic about activities that had once excited me. But Adrienne and I were taking two weeks off for the holidays: I thought I would be okay after that.

I love to read on holidays because it helps me switch off. So, as usual, I picked up a fiction book by an author I love. I just couldn't get into it. Thinking it was the book, I tried another; same outcome. I wasn't able to settle into my normal page-turning rhythm. I saw lines on a page but was not hearing a story. I went back over what I had just read, and it was as if I had not seen the words before. They had not registered. Was it my eyes? No, the page was not out of focus. I turned to videos that I had also stored up for the break. About ten minutes in, I fell asleep. This happened again and again. I chatted with Adrienne about what was happening. She told me that recently that usually happened when I watched TV. Oops! I was becoming bad company.

We came back from our holiday just in time for the birth of our first grandchild, Alexander. Holding my new grandson was joyful and profound, but the feeling of flatness and exhaustion remained underneath. I started looking for answers to change the way I was feeling. That winter, I remember a pastor friend ringing me to say that he'd been praying for me. He didn't know the stress I was under, but he could see something I couldn't. He asked, 'Don, where is your joy? Don't let anyone steal your joy.' I admitted that, yes, perhaps I had lost my joy but didn't see that I had become depressed. I should have taken this as a sign to talk to people who could help me. Instead, I just gritted my teeth and carried on.

Towards the end of January, I took time out for my quarterly "Prayer and Vision"— withdrawing for a few days, praying and reflecting on my work. While it is not a holiday, I usually return reinvigorated and energised by my time with God. This year, though, I had nothing left in the tank. I didn't do much praying, but I did sleep a lot. Blindly and lacking understanding of how sick I was, I wrongly self-scripted medicine to fix the problem: praying harder, working harder, and going harder at the gym.

I continued praying for an hour a day by my pool early in the morning. The pool was still and clear, but my spirit was in turmoil and clouded. My prayer was intense, driven and demanding. There was little sense of God's presence or peace. I was not talking with someone I felt close to; the conversation was from a desperate person grasping for things in an effort to improve their sense of well-being. I call this kind of prayer "adrenaline prayer."

I felt a need to exercise more, so I increased my gym activity. I yearned for the endorphins released in exercise. The pumping music of the gym and the loud push of the spin class instructor to climb higher and put in more effort made me feel good. It reinforced my belief that I was doing what I needed to do. The adrenaline kept pumping, and the blindness to impending burnout remained.

I took on more and more at work. I scheduled more meetings, made more phone calls, and preached with greater intensity. This intensity kept the adrenaline pumping, so it was so difficult to stop when I came to the end of the day. I constantly felt a tightness in my chest and wondered if it was a serious physical problem. That was when I first booked a doctor's appointment.

In preparing for the visit and thinking about what I was going to say, I wrote a list of difficulties I was experiencing:

- I'm experiencing immense fatigue
- I feel drained
- My mental capacity is reduced
- My decision making is slow
- Foggy brain—I don't have my usual sharpness
- I frequently lose my concentration, wander in conversations, find myself asking, "What did you just say?"
- I feel tired all the time.
- I'm peopled out.
- I'm short and irritable.
- I just want to withdraw from people (My family with whom I am deeply connected came over, but I wanted to go to my room, shut the door, lay on my bed and watch a video).

During the doctor's visit, I asked him to do blood tests, sure that I had a disease or a virus. It didn't enter my head that it wasn't my physical but my mental health that wasn't right. I thought it might be Barmah Forest Disease, a mosquito-borne virus. Ten years previously, I had experienced similar chronic fatigue-like symptoms when I had this virus. My muscles hurt, with and without exercise, my lymph nodes were swollen and tender, and there was an overwhelming feeling of lethargy and weakness. The symptoms of Barmah Forest Disease usually returned when I had any virus like a common cold, for instance.

Considering all the factors, the doctor ordered the blood tests, but he could see what I could not. He told me, "I think you are approaching burnout, and you need to rest."

But I wasn't ready to hear that yet.

Physical Signs

We all know the benefit of hindsight, and it's true; in retrospect, you see what you didn't amid a situation. It wasn't until I was in recovery that I was able to look back and see specific indications that I was heading for trouble. My psychiatrist helped me discover many other symptoms I had been carrying without realising. Let me share a few early indicators of stress that I wish I had given more attention.

My mouth was often dry. My psychiatrist once asked me to recall a stressful situation. I remembered a time when I had to deal with a leader's bad behaviour, and in sensing the stress at the start of the meeting, I excused myself to fill my glass with water. I realised that my mouth gets parched when pressure increases. I have drunk reasonable amounts of water for years, but the increased need indicated increasing stress.

My right thigh often tightened and felt numb. My doctor sent me to a physiotherapist who asked me what bothered me most. I told her about my right thigh, sometimes feeling like pins and needles, occasionally numb to the touch. She asked if I remembered when it had first happened. I instantly recalled being a leader at an Easter Camp in 1980. I received news that a young man, whom many young people and I knew, had just been killed in a car accident. He had just turned 16 and gotten his driver's licence. As I spoke to the young people and encouraged them to trust an eternal God, my right thigh became taut. Since then, it has tightened in times of high stress.

I had an elevated heart rate. The physiotherapist asked me to spin on a bike to raise my heart rate to 120bpm, and consequently, I became more aware of my heart rate. One night, when having trouble sleeping, I realised I had an elevated heart rate. I knew the average resting rate was 60bmp, but I was shocked to discover palpitations—my heart was racing at 90bpm. All I had been doing in the past hour was lying on the bed, trying to sleep.

These signs are likely specific to me and how my body reacts to stress. Not everyone will experience these symptoms. However, I encourage you to look at your own physical symptoms of stress and make careful notes of when they occur. Often, our body reacts to stress before we mentally acknowledge the difficulty of a situation.

Entering the Danger Zone

Ignoring the advice from my doctor, I continued on the same trajectory. The problem intensified. I had built personal disciplines over a long period of life, like safety rails to keep me safe physically, emotionally and spiritually. But these safety rails began to lose their stability. I was losing resilience, self-moderation and self-control.

I would eat my usual portion of food but still felt hungry. I felt empty inside and ate more to fill me. I gained about 10 kilograms in weight.

My morning ritual includes espresso coffee, made from freshly ground beans, carefully tamped to achieve a deep crema. Yet after my usual amount for the day, I still wanted more.

I enjoy a glass or two of Shiraz (especially from McLaren Vale, South Australia). But after two drinks, I still felt thirsty. The third glass made my head feel quieter—it was the numbing effect of alcohol that I desired.

Massage was beneficial for my aching body. But after a good massage, I immediately thought and planned the next appointment. I found that I wanted more touch.

Movies I watched were more violent, explicit and intense.

My sleep pattern changed. Two or three times a week, I took about two hours to drift off to sleep. Then on other nights, I would be wide awake for a couple of hours in the middle of the night. Sleep evaded me in my bed, yet I would constantly fall asleep during a TV programme.

When I noticed that someone wanted to talk to me, my mind would quickly flick through a list of worst-case possibilities. I constantly fought a feeling of failure or thoughts of rejection. My mind was self-destructing, and my self-value was slipping lower and lower.

A binge craving grew in all areas of my life. Little seemed to satisfy the increasing unquenchable desires. Temptations in all areas of life seemed stronger. It was as if the lines on the road had disappeared. A feeling of danger grew in me, a sense that a crash was imminent. The guard rails that guided my morality and behaviour were loose and wouldn't keep me from going over the edge. I felt unsafe.

The Three Components of Burnout

My quest to understand burnout led me to the highly-credible Duke University study on burnout. In 2010, the Duke University launched the Duke Clergy Health Initiative funded by a large endowment. In their summary report, they acknowledge that burnout has three components: *"high emotional exhaustion, high depersonalisation, and low sense of personal accomplishment."* [8]

Their studies and research show that "Burnout, in its three-factor structure, is not just a potential problem to clergy but applies to occupations that are focused on helping people to live better lives. Occupations where people become engaged with people providing guidance, preventing harm, and helping people to do well, emotionally, cognitively or physically."[9] These occupations—teachers, nurses, doctors, social workers, health counsellors, therapists, police, EMTs, firefighters and the like—place staff at risk of burnout.

I want to take some time to dive a little deeper into these three components of burnout and how they first appeared in my life.

High Emotional Exhaustion

Seeing a psychologist was an integral step in my healing. It was not an immediate fix as my burnout was severe, but his clinical assessment

---

[8] Proeschold-Bell, Rae Jean, et al. *The Glory of God Is a Human Being Fully Alive: Predictors of Positive versus Negative Metal Health Fund among Clergy.* Duke University, https://divinity.duke.edu/sites/divinity.duke.edu/files/documents/chi/Predictors%20of%20positive%20versus%20negative%20mental%20health%20among%20clergy_web2.pdf

[9] Proeschold-Bell, Rae Jean, et al. The Glory of God Is a Human Being Fully Alive: Predictors of Positive versus Negative Metal Health Fund among Clergy. Duke University, https://divinity.duke.edu/sites/divinity.duke.edu/files/documents/chi/Predictors%20of%20positive%20versus%20negative%20mental%20health%20among%20clergy_web2.pdf

helped correct my self-diagnosis and self-prescription. He gave me a test to diagnose my condition, measuring my depression, anxiety and stress. The diagnosis was as follows: Stress: High, Anxiety: Moderate, Depression: Mild. I was surprised by the outcome. Me? Mild depression? Moderate anxiety? Yes, I knew I was stressed, but I was surprised that it was at a dangerously high level.

As we chatted in the sessions over the following weeks, it became apparent my emotional tank had run dry. I kept thinking about the rainwater tank in our old house. Living in the world's driest continent, catching rainwater is valuable, mainly because we pay for every litre we consume. An electric motor, which started when a tap was turned on, pumped water from the tank to the house.

Occasionally, there would be no flow of water. My first thought was always that something was wrong with the pump, or a tap was turned off at the tank, but I could hear the pump running and running. Yet water wasn't flowing. The first time this happened, I went outside to the pump. I placed my hand on it. It was scalding and made much more noise than usual. When I tapped the tank, it sounded hollow at every rung to the ground. I climbed the ladder to look inside and found it empty. So, I turned off the motor, letting it rest, and waited for rain to fill the tank. Fortunately, we were able to turn on the mains water while we waited for rain. After a tropical downpour filled the tank, I switched the rainwater system back on, and rainwater flowed from the tank out the tap.

Running constantly while being emotionally empty had caused me to feel faulty. Like thinking the problem of the rainwater was the pump, I thought I was the problem; that I was broken, rather than dried up.

Was I empty simply because I had not been filling the tank? I would have once said, "No!" very strongly. In my endeavour to just keep pumping to make the water flow, I worked hard at "keeping the tank full", but I was blind to the structural problems in my life and the damage sustained over thirty-eight years of ministry. My psychologist was like the ladder I needed to help me look down into my emotional tank. He helped me see it was empty, and the holes in my emotional tank led to perceptions and responses that could (and had) caused harm. Emotionally, I had no more to give.

High detachment from team and people

In the initial list of my symptoms, I noted that I was "peopled out," but it was not evident that I was becoming detached from my team, friends, and even family. I was short and irritable and just wanted to withdraw. I did not understand that this is part of burnout; it wasn't how I had imagined detachment to feel. Rather, I imagined I was building a safety zone around my world to keep away from negative emotional impacts.

One of the apparent signs was that I did not settle in conversation. When I was chatting with someone, I constantly looked past them, seeing whom I would talk to next. I thought that I was engaged but sent the opposite signal. Detachment from my team and people had been increasing for some time before my condition was diagnosed.

The holes in my emotional tank, the lack of trust and feelings of rejection finally made me step back from people. It was both scary and safe; scary as I didn't want to be like that, yet safe in that I wouldn't be harmed. I felt internal conflict.

I began to anticipate the worst in my work and team. When a team member rang, my mind played an internal script of condemnation and rejection. I started fearing people would leave. I expected them to bring bad news, even though that was not usually the outcome of the calls or communication. The emotional depletion I was experiencing was feeding the increasing detachment. I became fearful, anxious and avoidant.

God designed us to have healthy attachments in our key relationships;

marriage, family, friends and work teams. In speaking of marriage, Arch Hart and Sharon Morris acknowledge four attachment types in the book *Safe Haven Marriage*[10]. "Four attachment styles have been identified, and a proper understanding of them is essential to building a safe haven marriage: secure, anxious, avoidant, and fearful (which, in children, is identified as disorganised/ambivalent)."

A helpful resource to understand emotional intelligence and, in particular, its integration with our key relationships is the book by Bradberry and Greaves; *Emotional Intelligence 2.0*.[11] Bradberry and Greaves identify four skills in emotional intelligence; self-awareness, self-management, social awareness and relationship management. "Self-awareness is your ability to accurately perceive your own emotions in the moment and understand your tendencies across situations." As my emotional tank became depleted, it became much harder to self-manage my emotions.[12] Bradberry and Greaves say, "Self-management is your ability to use your awareness of your emotions to stay flexible and direct your behaviour positively."[13] I lacked empathy

---

10 Hart, Archibald; Morris, Sharon. *Safe Haven Marriage*. Thomas Nelson. Kindle Edition.(p. 70)

11 Talent Smart 2009

12 Bradberry and Greaves "Emotional Intelligence 2.0" Talent Smart 2009

13 Bradberry and Greaves "Emotional Intelligence 2.0" Talent Smart 2009

for others; I didn't listen in conversations and became easily agitated with people. With my self-management diminished, it's not surprising that social awareness plummeted. Bradberry and Greaves add that "Social awareness is your ability to accurately pick up on emotions in other people and understand what is really going on with them."[14] Instead of seeing the pain in others' emotions, I would take their comments personally. It's no wonder that low self-awareness, low self-management, and low social awareness result in inadequate relationship management. Bradberry and Greaves complete their list with, "Relationship management is your ability to use your awareness of your own emotions and those of others to manage interactions successfully. This ensures clear communication and effective handling of conflict."[15] When conflict arose, I tended to avoid the problems.

So, the increasing detachment added to the emotional depletion. Thankfully, the converse is true; good relationships replenish our emotions.

Low satisfaction with work

The high emotional depletion and the increasing sense of detachment

---

14 Bradberry and Greaves "Emotional Intelligence 2.0" Talent Smart 2009

15 Bradberry and Greaves "Emotional Intelligence 2.0" Talent Smart 2009

gave me a rising dissatisfaction with my work. My tank drained more, the sighs deepened, frustration with people increased, detachment increased, all making me feel worse. I was lacking in energy, and the thought of the new year didn't fill me with hope and life. I felt more trapped and powerless to effect change. I can relate to the Rolling Stones when they say they "can't get no satisfaction"!

I had always had a strong sense of what I was doing and why. It felt wrong to feel so lost, exhausted and discouraged while doing God's work. In the article, *"The Glory of God is a Human Being Fully Alive"*[16], the writers assert that a feeling of calling may actually drive workers to behaviours that can result in burnout.

"Like clergy, many caregiving professionals feel called to their work, even if their call is derived from a desire to help others and a feeling that one's work is making a difference rather than a desire to serve God. As noted above, attributing a higher meaning to one's work increases the stakes of both failure and success and may drive workers to behaviours that result in burnout and contribute to depression and anxiety."[17]

---

16 Proeschold-Bell, Rae Jean, et al. The Glory of God Is a Human Being Fully Alive: Predictors of Positive versus Negative Metal Health Fund among Clergy. Duke University

17 Stalker et al. 2007

For me, this was true. I kept thinking, *I'm serving God, so why is this not working?* My conclusion was, "I am the problem." This impacted my identity and sense of self-worth; I began to think I was no good and unable to produce anything.

How did I get to this place?

Burnout results from too much stress for too long, but that doesn't necessarily address the real reason that some people burn out. My psychologist was able to help me see the root of the problem with one simple question: "Why do you place such a low value on yourself?"

I won't speak for everyone who has reached burnout; I'm sure many paths lead to an empty tank, but I would imagine that low self-value is a common cause. People who value themselves and their wellness don't run themselves into the ground. There is almost always a psychological reason. Some people push themselves out of pride, some from a desire to help, some from avoidance of other aspects of life. Often, there are multiple reasons, but it usually comes down to the fact that they are putting too many things above their well-being.

My psychologist probed around self-image: How do I see myself? Why do I push myself so hard without stopping to revive? Ultimately, I had put a high value on my career, success and other people in my life, and the fact that I refused to slow down and rest showed that I had placed a low value on myself and my needs.

I had been known as a person of strong resilience all my working life. When I encountered difficulties, I could bounce back in no time at all. My sense of worth was linked to hard work. I had an over-realised sense of responsibility. I felt it was my place to make everything right: that I would carry more weight in the load, that it was my duty to pay more. My early Christian worldview taught me to self-empty as Jesus did. "(He) emptied himself, by taking the form of a servant, being born in the likeness of men."[18] Unlike Jesus, I thought I could just continue without replenishing. I had a proper Protestant work ethic; diligence, discipline and hard work were the keys to success.[19] I thought that time to replenish would be pandering to my vanity. Many highly-driven people, used to taking problems in stride, can feel a failure when admitting they are overwhelmed, stressed, tired and in need. I realised my self-image had blinded me to my actual needs.

---

18 Philippians 2:7 ESV

19 https://www.britannica.com/topic/Protestant-ethic

In many ways, burnout is the symptom of addiction to hard work, people-pleasing and adrenaline. As with any addiction, the first step is recognising that you have a problem.

Technology and burnout

Unequivocally, technology contributed to my burnout, not as the primary cause, but as a dangerous additive—like rain making the road slippery so that a crash is more likely in wet weather.

I can see now that I had become addicted to my smartphone. It was my constant companion, going everywhere I went, enabling me to be online 24/7. I prided myself on responding to emails within an hour of receiving them, except when I slept. I would check my emails and messages and respond within a short space of waking. The last thing I would do at night was check my emails and messages and respond. Smart technology has changed everything about how we work; we no longer need to be in an office or even on a computer to get things done; we can work from almost anywhere. This development makes creating healthy work/life boundaries much more complicated than it used to be. I find it fascinating that the German Labour Ministry has banned out-of-office hours working, following on from similar restrictions on out-of-hours emails imposed by German firms including Volkswagen, BMW, and Puma[20] in the attempt to limit the pressure to be connected at all times.

Emails were only a part of my problem. Facebook, Twitter, Instagram had me hooked. I was constantly looking for that post that mentioned me. Some get depressed as they use Facebook, some get addicted, and some both. I became addicted. Arch Hart's brilliant book *The Digital Invasion: How Technology is Shaping You and Your Relationships* cites *Psychology Today* saying that Facebook and Twitter are more addictive than tobacco and alcohol. Hart addresses the impact of technology on our relationships by giving current research into the links between social media and emotional well-being. The fear of missing out and Facebook depression are becoming clinical terms.

The key to health is management of the addiction. Six months of abstaining and then only limited use assisted my health journey. I still have not gone back to Facebook or Twitter and have recently stopped using Instagram again because I found some of the posts I saw messed with me emotionally. I remember seeing someone riding a Harley when I couldn't afford one. I knew I should be just happy for them,

---

20 Vasagar, Jeevan. "Out of Hours WORKING Banned by German Labour Ministry." *The Telegraph*, Telegraph Media Group, 30 Aug. 2013,
www.telegraph.co.uk/news/worldnews/europe/germany/10276815/Out-of-hours-working-banned-by-German-labour-ministry.html.

but all I felt was disappointment with myself for not measuring up to this person I barely knew. Once again, I was fighting feelings of missing out and failure. So, I hit delete!

I feel some grief in not being as virtually connected to my global friends. These are people that I have spent meaningful time with face-to-face and have only limited time with now. So, I have learned to smile as I recall great friends and treasure the times we have spent together, rather than pandering to my insecurities in looking for acknowledgement. I know they appreciate me without posting a message on Facebook for the world to see. Let's build a world where we can trust each other at our word.

Adrienne wears a silver locket given to my mum's grandmother, Sarah, by her fiancé William on their engagement in Yorkshire, England. William set sail for Australia in the late 1800s, saying, "I will send for you when things are ready." Three years later, Sarah received a letter, "Come now." The boat carrying the letter took three months to arrive. Over six months after William sent word, Sarah arrived. They were married the next day. William kept his word, "I will send for you." Sarah kept her word, "I will come." Through remaining true to their word, William and Sarah built a strong foundation of trust in their relationship.

Today, Sarah would have face-timed William, as she travelled to Heathrow, instant messaged as she passed customs, faced-timed in Dubai, or mid-air depending on the class of her ticket, iMessaged when she landed. He would have been tracking her plane's flight progress. Does the quantum leap in communication help our relational well-being? The statistics say no. Marriages are more at risk now. Enhanced communication access is not the fault, but often it's used to prop up our insecurities brought about by the changeability of our word and disposable relationships. It can make our communication and expression of feelings seem shallow by their frequency, questioning and thoughtlessness. Texts driven by insecurities can build insecurity. My tip is to ensure that socials are affirming and encouraging. Ask yourself, what will they hear in my message? The adage "think before you speak" applies here. Think before you hit send.

Technology is a tool. It is not evil in itself, but it can cause great harm when not used in the right way. We must use it with care; rule it, not be ruled by it. I love woodworking. I built the mantle shelf for a fireplace in our new home using timber from a red gum tree that we had to remove to build the house. The shelf is mitred at the front ends. The mitre cut was tricky to do on a drop saw, as the timber is thicker than the depth of cut and needed placing in four different ways to complete it. And I still have all my fingers, unlike the person I purchased the saw from a couple of years ago! Tools can be dangerous; that shouldn't prohibit their use. They just require safety measures to be applied.

Likewise, my journey has caused me to apply safety measures to my use of digital technology. Do you have a management plan for technology? When do you respond to emails? When do you access social media? Dr Sylvia Hart Frejd encourages the setting of digital boundaries[21]. I especially love the boundary of no digital gadgets at mealtimes. Be present at the table. Let's have real conversations with real people! I find the number of couples at a restaurant both on their phones during most of the meal disturbing. Leave the phone in the car and if you need to be contacted by the babysitter go old-school and give them the restaurant number. My emotional tank is healthier when I build relationships by being present and not being distracted by my iPhone.

The answer to the technology dilemma is moderation not abstinence. The real goal here is to be present with the people around you, or sometimes just present with yourself. We all want to enjoy the world as we interact with it, and we want to enjoy the company of those with

---

21 "Love Enough to Set Limits on Using Digital Devices"

Hart, Dr. Archibald D.; Hart Frejd, Dr. Sylvia. The Digital Invasion: How Technology is Shaping You and Your Relationships (p. 171). Baker Publishing Group. Kindle Edition.

us. This is easier without the bings and buzzes reminding you of everything outside your current situation. You'll find you miss so much less and enjoy so much more when your phone is tucked away and only brought out at intentional times.

As a parent, friend and pastor, I teach responsibility rather than prohibition. Prohibition breeds rebellion, whereas responsibility seeds self-control—and may at times mean abstaining. So, with social media, I promote responsibility. Technology is a wonderful tool. Let's use it wisely to enhance our well-being.

The Danger of Wrong Self-prescriptions

Before coming to terms with my burnout and taking the advice of my general practitioner, I thought I could fix it myself. I am a firm believer that I partner with God in the outcomes of life, but I was not partnering with Him nor the people He had given me to help my well-being. Not only had I self-diagnosed the problem, but also, I self-prescribed my medication: a short holiday.

The solutions I was applying were not wrong but used at the wrong time. Holidays are great and necessary, but they do not always fix the problems of impending burnout. I was seriously sick and needed extended rest as well as a significant change to my lifestyle. After the holiday, I was returning to work to the same work patterns and behaviours that contributed to burnout.

There are activities that are vital for both a healthy lifestyle and success under normal circumstances—however, those change with burnout. Intense prayer and retreats, hard work, and spending ample time with peers and family are necessary to my overall mental health, and I thought they would help me in this time of depletion. However, they were not the solution—they even got in the way of what I truly needed: rest. Now I look back and feel as if I was trying to fix a broken leg with exercise.

In February, my GP again said, *'You are approaching burnout.'* By now, I understood what I was feeling wasn't normal. Yet it was some time before I realised the severity of my condition. I stubbornly kept pushing on while planning to take time off from April. The GP offered me some medication—he called them "happy pills"—to balance my emotions. We agreed that initially, I would seek help from the psychologist and review the possibility of medication later.

Please call it what it is: Burnout

Admitting you are sick means you know you need to get well. As with finding directions on a map to the place you want to go, you need to know your location first.

Adrienne is a tutor. She tutors literacy and numeracy, mostly to primary and secondary students. She has also had the pleasure of teaching a man in his 30's to read. Still, she could only start to teach him after he stopped hiding his disability. When he felt safe enough to acknowledge, "I can't read," he was able to be offered gratis help to learn. What a beautiful moment it was when he said to the other guys in our small group, "Tonight, I am going to read from the Bible." We need safe communities to transparently share our problems and receive the help we need without judgement.

If I were to acknowledge my difficulties, I thought I would be talking myself into a worse situation. But ignoring the symptoms of burnout only made them worse. I am not alone in living in denial of burnout; I watched some of my colleagues try to work around it instead of admitting they were sick. I've known people who have decided to take a sabbatical amid burnout, thinking that a change of location or focus will solve their problem. Sabbatical is a time for learning and discovery, not storing energy and revitalising. When my friends returned home, they felt just as exhausted, and this was made worse by their colleagues pressuring them to share their new insights. My friends needed to admit they were burnt out and accept a proper break from everything work-related so they could recover.

If you benefit from working with peers and an overseer, it's to your immense benefit to be transparent with how you are actually doing. Not only are they able to help in recognising a difficulty, but they can also significantly assist in finding solutions. I discovered that acknowledging my struggle to those I work with helped lessen my emotional load.

Being clear and upfront about your struggles also helps others facing difficulty with burnout. Hiding your pain reinforces the huge negative stigma attached to emotional problems. Bringing burnout into the light through candid conversation gives others the permission and courage to do something about it, helping to stop the propensity to withdraw in shame. I was pleasantly surprised to have others say to me, "I have been where you are." My admission permitted them to disclose their own experience.

If you find yourself identifying with the symptoms I describe, please get professional help. Visit your GP. See a psychologist. I know that it can be difficult, and pride can get in the way (especially for males!). Be courageous and vulnerable and talk about how you truly are. I encourage you not to deny your journey but call it what it is.

Walking with a limp

Jacob was a man who followed after his grandfather, Abraham, and his father, Isaac, by putting his faith in God. There is one particular story about him that I like to sit with now: the story of Jacob wrestling God found in Genesis 32:22-31 (NLT).

> *[22] During the night, Jacob got up and took his two wives, his two servant wives, and his eleven sons and crossed the Jabbok River with them. [23] After taking them to the other side, he sent over all his possessions.*
>
> *[24] This left Jacob all alone in the camp, and a man came and wrestled with him until the dawn began to break. [25] When the man saw that he would not win the match, he touched Jacob's hip and wrenched it out of its socket. [26] Then the man said, "Let me go, for the dawn is breaking!"*
>
> *But Jacob said, "I will not let you go unless you bless me."*
>
> *[27] "What is your name?" the man asked.*
>
> *He replied, "Jacob."*
>
> *[28] "Your name will no longer be Jacob," the man told him. "From now on you will be called Israel, because you have fought*

> *with God and with men and have won."*
> *²⁹ "Please tell me your name," Jacob said.*
> *"Why do you want to know my name?" the man replied. Then he blessed Jacob there.*
> *³⁰ Jacob named the place Peniel ("face of God"), for he said, "I have seen God face to face, yet my life has been spared."*
> *³¹ The sun was rising as Jacob left Peniel, and he was limping because of the injury to his hip.*

This is such a profound metaphor for burnout. The wrestling birthed a change in Jacob's identity—God changed his name to Israel—his strength shifted, and in the end, he became the man God created him to be. Isaiah 43: 1-3 is written to Jacob/Israel, addressing what this change in him meant:

> *But now, O Jacob, listen to the Lord who created you.*
> *O Israel, the one who formed you says,*
> *"Do not be afraid, for I have ransomed you.*
> *I have called you by name; you are mine.*
> *² When you go through deep waters,*
> *I will be with you.*
> *When you go through rivers of difficulty,*
> *you will not drown.*

When you walk through the fire of oppression,
you will not be burned up;
the flames will not consume you.
³ For I am the Lord, your God,
the Holy One of Israel, your Saviour."

It begins by reminding God's children of Jacob and his name change to Israel. It says Jacob listened to the Lord, his creator. It reminds us not to be afraid for God is with us through difficulties. I love this passage because it reminds me that God created me, and more than that, he formed my identity like steel is formed in the furnace—with heat and pressure. These difficulties that I've walked and will walk through are there for my formation.

As with Jacob/Israel, who walked with a limp afterwards, going through struggles does affect us. But I say this as encouragement; you will also come out wiser and more robust in other ways. For me, some things are not the same and never will be. I tire more easily. I'm far more aware of my humanity, vulnerability, weakness, but I am also more aware of my strengths and purpose. While you are in burnout, have faith that you will grow from the experience. You might even look back in the years to come and find yourself grateful you went through this hardship. I know that I am.

Reflection Questions for Chapter Two

1) Are there signs that I am dealing with any of the three components of burnout?

- Emotional exhaustion
- Detachment from people
- Dissatisfaction with work

2) What are my symptoms? Make a list.

3) When did I last chat with my GP about my emotional wellbeing? How honest was I with what I said?

CHAPTER 3

Recovery: Rest & Replenishment

After the Crash

There is good news. You can get better!

There is an increasing sense of helplessness in the journey towards burnout. It's like hitting water on the road, losing traction, and the ABS failing to kick in. It seems that nothing you do makes a difference, and you have lost control. You turn the steering wheel this way or that, and it makes no difference. You reach for the brake, but it has no effect. The slide continues. Adrenaline is pumping through your body, everything is going fast, yet it seems like you are watching your slide in slow motion.

Then the crash. You realise you are stationary. Everything seems blurry. You feel numb as the body self-medicates the pain. There is a relief that the slide has stopped, but also, there is assessment of injury and damage. Will this vehicle go again? Can I get to my destination?

For me, the crash was soon after coming home from my holiday and recognising that I was not rested from my break. I was more numb and more exhausted than ever.

There is a verse in Psalm 1:3 that talks of flourishing:

> *They are like trees planted along the riverbank,*
> *bearing fruit each season.*
> *Their leaves never wither,*
> *and they prosper in all they do.*

I was like a tree that had become sick and wondered if I could ever again be a picture of vibrant life, producing fruit? I felt the opposite of that tree.

Stop, Revive, Survive

As a twenty-two-year-old, I recall making a six-hour journey at night from a concert to the place I was living in the South-East of South Australia. About two hours into the trip, I began to feel very weary. I turned up the music I had bought at the concert, drank Coke, ate chocolate and wound down the window letting the cold air fill the car. But I was feeling more and more sleepy. I finally realised that I was failing the fight against sleep, so I pulled over, stopped the car and got out. The exhaustion seemed to engulf me. Stopping seemed to make it worse, but really, stopping just allowed me to realise how tired I was. So, I sat in the car and slept. I awoke refreshed and continued my journey safely.

On the highway from Queensland to Sydney, you will often see Stop, Revive, Survive signs on the side of the road in Northern New South Wales. Their purpose is to reduce road fatality; driver fatigue is one of the three major killers on NSW roads, so the government implemented a "driver reviver" programme of education and application. The signs are an indicator that a rest stop is just ahead. There are now over 80 sites where over 5000 volunteers serve two quintessential Australian icons: Bushels tea and Arnott's biscuits.[22] Regular reviver stops are necessary to survive a long car trip. This is also true emotionally. Stopping is essential; if you don't revive, you become fatigued, which is extremely dangerous for your survival.

Stop, Revive, Survive could be the mantra for burnout recovery. While I had ceased work, I took some time to come to a complete stop: the severity of my burnout had a momentum of its own. I call this part of the journey "going through the valley of depletion."

---

22 http://roadsafety.transport.nsw.gov.au/stayingsafe/fatigue/driverreviver/index.html

The Valley of Depletion

I did not improve at the moment I ceased work. On the contrary, I seemed to get worse. With each passing week, I became more aware of my depletion.

In the last chapter, I talked about how my psychologist helped me become more aware of the symptoms of being depleted, like dryness in my mouth when I was anxious, which continued into my recovery. Likewise, my palms would sweat, sometimes my hands would shake, and my shoulders would get tense when stressed. I was still dealing with intense physical symptoms of my burnout. The dynamo running inside took some time to slow. A friend of mine played in the Australian Football League competition. After a night game, he said it would take about 4 hours for the adrenaline to slow down enough to get some sleep. For me, after years of running on adrenaline, I needed months for it to stop.

Two months into the time off, Adrienne and I went to Sydney to visit our daughter and her husband, who had recently moved there. Typically, I take charge of travel arrangements. If we travelled on a bus, I would look up where to get on and get off. This time I said to Adrienne, "You need to work out which bus we are catching and tell me when to get off. Sorry, I just can't do it."

Permission to rest

Even though burnout has only recently become a normalised topic of discussion, it has been around since people could feel stress—forever! Even Biblical prophets experienced burnout. The prophet Elijah suffered from it after Jezebel chased him into the wilderness. Alone and fearing for his life, Elijah found a cave to hide. He was dissatisfied with his work and depressed. Elijah wasn't doing anything wrong, and he wasn't being idle. Instead, he had been focused on a difficult assignment for a long time—he was just depleted. He called to God, "I have zealously served the Lord God Almighty. But the people of Israel have broken their covenant with you, torn down your altars, and killed every one of your prophets. I am the only one left, and now they are trying to kill me, too."[23] He felt that he was the only one left doing God's work, and he had nothing left to give.

I identify with this story, not only because of how relatable Elijah was in this situation but because of God's response. God sent angels to minister to Elijah and bring him replenishment. He allowed Elijah to rest and recover while reminding him that he wasn't alone. After rest and God's encouragement, Elijah returned to his work with his assignment clarified and a larger sense of purpose. He went on to

---

23 1 Kings 19:10 (NLT)

mentor Elisha to continue his work. God allows us to rest.

For years, I used a prioritised task list to help me be productive. But in stopping, I no longer had a list of things to be completed. My task list app stayed closed, and I turned off all alerts and reminders. I kept saying to myself, "Today, Don, your task is to rest so you can get well." I started taking naps during the day. I would sleep two to three hours during the afternoon and be surprised that I still slept at night.

Even though I was resting, I was frustrated that I only felt worse. My brain was foggier, the thought processes harder. I could not handle crowds, especially if I were not close to an exit. Noise was overwhelming. Even going to the shopping mall was hard work. It was safer to just stay at home. I would walk 100 meters and then need to lay down and rest. The tangibles that I began to see showed me I was still declining.

My doctor said that adrenal fatigue was kicking in. Now that I had ceased to run on adrenaline, my body was reacting. Everything was catching up to me. Did I get worse because I stopped? No. It was like that night when I was twenty-two and stepped out of the car only to realise how exhausted I truly was. My body was showing me just how much I needed this rest. Partly, I was becoming more aware of the impact of fatigue on my body, and secondly, my body was responding to the permission to rest after finally acknowledging my illness. The deep problems were working their way out like a deeply embedded splinter, and as with a splinter, I felt the difficulties more acutely as they surfaced. And when the splinter is out, relief and healing follow.

Replenishing Activities

As the months progressed, I started to see some lift in the exhaustion I felt. I took up woodworking. I had the opportunity to purchase two cubic metres of silky oak, rough-sawn timber. I milled it at a friend's workshop to make it ready for fine furniture-making. I designed and built a sofa table, carefully joining the timbers for the top and mitring the legs. The further I got with the project, the more satisfaction it gave me. I woke in the mornings with excitement to continue the project, and as I lay on the bed at night, I would think of the next thing to do. Once I began to feel some energy again, doing something productive and creative with my time was important. I was starting to feel a bounce in my step again.

The things that had ceased to bring me joy for the last year became fun and stimulating once again. I've always loved taking walks and riding my motorbike; finally, I found these exercises cathartic and exciting. I could read books without getting antsy; I could watch movies without falling asleep.

Also, I noticed that I wanted to spend more time with people instead of withdrawing or avoiding. I began to feel more and more attached to the ones I love. A simple dinner with my family made me feel so happy and grateful for their presence and support and seeing friends I hadn't seen in a long time filled me with joy. In the process of filling the tank and replenishing the emotions, there is nothing like time with loved ones; time with my wife, my children, their spouses, the grandkids—nothing fills the tank like that.

It is now known that good relationships are vital for good mental health and affect how long we live. Dan Siegel, author of *The Developing Mind* says, "Relationships are the key factor associated with medical and mental health, longevity, and even happiness."[24] Given that relationships are vital for us to flourish, it is imperative that we guard ourselves against the competing activities of our culture and deliberately invest in time with our loved ones. Simple things like eating together, talking together, building healthy, secure relationships make a big difference. Stephen Covey the author of the *7 Habits of Highly Effective People* is reported to say,

---

24. Dr Dan Siegel, The Developing Mind Second EditionHow Relationships and the Brain Interact to Shape Who We Are.

"I think the most significant work we'll do in our whole life, in our whole world, is done within the four walls of our home." [25]

Working on my relationships and finding them secure after feeling detachment for so long, was a true blessing. Not only had my friends and family helped me through my burnout when I had become bad company, but also, through the recovery process. They were so patient with me, and I am truly grateful.

Crucial Recovery Roles

I want to take a moment to recognise a significant help for those going through emotional difficulties; that is other people. No one can get through burnout alone. Here, I want to acknowledge those around me who supported and helped me through my recovery.

Friends

Friends can be a strong help. As I've acknowledged, I had little understanding of emotional difficulties before my burnout. If I sensed someone was signalling to be left alone, I would walk away, assuming they didn't need or want help. As I look back, I can see some people I was involved with were not coping well emotionally. I'm embarrassed

---

[25] The Wisdom and Teachings of Stephen R. Covey

to say I misread the situation in many of these instances, and I took the lack of communication, the agitation, the withdrawal personally. I'm so sorry.

The reason I'm saying this is because, during the darkest times, a couple of my friends said, *"Don, you will get through this."* At first, these words seemed so faint and distant. It was as if I had shifted realities and slipped into another dimension. As my friends' words travelled to my numb and isolated land, they attached themselves securely to my heart and began pulling me back to health. Their calm voices made me feel so peaceful. The voice resonating in my spirit assured me. My friends were a living example of 2 Corinthians 1:3-5 from the New Living Translation:

> *[3] All praise to God, the Father of our Lord Jesus Christ. God is our merciful Father and the source of all comfort. [4] He comforts us in all our troubles so that we can comfort others. When they are troubled, we will be able to give them the same comfort God has given us. [5] For the more we suffer for Christ, the more God will shower us with his comfort through Christ.*

Others' pain, their experience of difficulty and consequent healing equipped them to help me. So, thanks to my mates who spoke words of encouragement to me. I'm so grateful.

Here is something that I can now pass on to others experiencing burnout: if you've been through difficult times like I'm talking about, the comfort you have received has equipped you to comfort others.

A note for the friends of those in recovery:

High detachment is a component of burnout that can be very hard to understand, both for those experiencing it and those outside. If you know a friend going through burnout, you have probably felt hurt and perhaps angry as the effort they once put into your relationship is now gone. In the same way, as it is hard to offer comfort to a person in grief when you've had no experience of suffering, it is also not easy to provide support for those with mental/emotional difficulties. It can be easy to take it personally when they don't answer the phone, when they avoid engaging, and when they pull away. Even as your mate begins to recover, they might still seek solitude and rest. Trust me; it's not you—it's the sickness.

People tend to react in one of two ways when they feel a friend detaching. Some will insist that they spend time together; they will attempt to engage and help in any way possible. Yet, the more they push in, the more the friend pulls away because this isn't what they need. It can be hard to let go, but they will return and engage again. Right now, they need the space to rest.

The other reaction is to withdraw. Because of hurt or discomfort, some people cannot engage with someone experiencing burnout. They don't know what to do, so they do nothing. They might even convince themselves that this is what their friend wants—just to be left alone.

What mates in recovery need is something in the middle of these two reactions. They need both space and encouragement. Small affirmations—even just a text or a voicemail—can mean the world. In these times, as in moments of grief, cliche statements don't cut it; honesty wins the day.

My strong encouragement here is that you stick by your mates. Try not to take things personally, rather be consistent in your connection and secure in who you are. Linger long enough to find out what's going on but give space when it's clear they are overwhelmed. Let's encourage one another with these words, *"You are going to get through this."*

I'm so grateful for the friends who stuck by me through my period of detachment without smothering or expecting me to perform in ways I couldn't. My true friends endured and were also integral in the process of re-attaching.

One of the many wooden things I've made is a chopping board with laminated pieces of timber glued alongside each other. Each thin piece of wood on its own will bend and lose its shape, but laminated together with others, each piece, and consequently, the board stays flat and sturdy. Ecclesiastes 4:12 says: *"Though one may be overpowered, two can defend themselves. A cord of three strands is not quickly broken."* Finding people you can rely on, join with, to help build attachment again is a necessary part of the strengthening, healing process.

Mentors

Just over twelve months into the journey back to health, I listened to a man called Keith Farmer address the national leadership of our C3 Church. He spoke about the value of a sabbatical for helping ministers to maintain good emotional vitality. I was fascinated by what Keith was saying. He had been where I had emotionally and was now focused on building mentoring relationships to help ministers flourish and experience wholeness. After chatting with Keith privately, he agreed to mentor me to help me eventually help others.

As we met over the next couple of years, Keith kept asking me questions, covering the most important aspects of my life.

My spirituality: How are you doing spiritually? How is your vitality in your relationship with Jesus?

My relationships: How are you and Adrienne? How are things with the children? The grandchildren? How are things with the team at work?

My emotional tank: Where would you place yourself on a scale of 0 to 10, with zero being "There's no way I can get out of bed today" and ten being "I'm ready to take on the whole world"?

My general lifestyle/health: What is your sleep pattern like? Are you having a consistent day off? What are you doing that is fun? How often are you exercising? (These are about sustainability.)

My places of risk: How are you doing with this personal vice (like alcohol)? What's happening now? How are you going with your diet? (I had mentioned I wanted to lose weight)

If the devil was going to take you out, how would he do it? (A way of checking in on my spiritual health and personal vices.)

I so valued this fatherly relationship. Keith's calm voice and affirming words made me feel settled, solid and secure. I felt heard, valued and encouraged through our time together, and my emotional tank filled.

Over thirty-seven years of ministry, I made many mistakes. I promoted the wrong people. I had not paid off enough debt and spent too much cash flow on operations. I had not fired people when they deserved to be sacked. I'd been too nice, putting up with slackness. I failed to give time for professional development after completing my Doctor of

Ministry in 1992. I'd not given myself time for personal hobbies. But the biggest mistake of all was not looking after my emotional health. I now see that a mentor could have helped me see some of my failings early on. They could have helped me avoid depletion. My firm conviction is that a mentoring relationship solely focused on how I am doing emotionally would have made a big difference.

Rick Lewis, in his book *Mentoring Matters,* says that one of the key values of a mentor is that they can see what you can't see[26], and that reflective feedback by the mentor can help a mentee to discover what they do not see.

A mentor can also help us discover our purpose. For example, my mentor Keith Farmer encouraged me to take a sabbatical. A sabbatical is different from long-service leave, which is to restore the soul. A sabbatical is to gain new skills and knowledge. Thanks to Keith, I was able to travel again to Fuller Theological Seminary and sit in a doctoral class titled "The Health of a Leader." The experience was valuable because it helped to identify my areas of passion. Understanding what lights you up, what gets you out of bed, is very empowering. This clarity enables us to be discriminatory with our time use—to know

---

26 Rick Lewis, Mentoring Matters, page 183ff

where to say *yes* and where to say *no*. Where once we may have operated out of a pleasing-others mentality, we now understand God's purpose for us, and hence where passion flows through us so that we work to please Him.

Monique Valcour, in The Harvard Business Review, commented on beating burnout; "The best antidote to burnout, particularly when it's driven by cynicism and inefficacy, is seeking out rich interpersonal interactions and continual personal and professional development. Find coaches and mentors who can help you identify and activate positive relationships and learning opportunities."[27]

Psychologists

Walking through the door to visit a psychologist was one of the hardest things I have done. The stigma of mental illness was still strong in my mind, but I knew by then that my pride was hurting me.

It took me about three months of visits to trust, listen and rest, months of visits to realise this was a safe place. I needed time for it to sink into my soul that my weaknesses would not be exposed to the world. Through my psychologist, I saw just how emotionally depleted I was and that resting could restore me. As the sessions progressed, I turned a

---

[27] Harvard Business Review, Monique Valcour. November 2016 issue.

corner and began to feel hope and purpose.

I recall many sessions with my psychologist, who constantly affirmed me. He would often say, "Don, if you did nothing else, what you have accomplished is wonderful." As I began to heal, he challenged me with questions like, "What is your purpose? What do you want to achieve?" I talked about wanting to change people's lives. He pushed me further in this, "Why have you been doing what you were doing?" I told him what I had always felt was true: God called me to connect people to him. But as I said this, I felt a sense of failure and that I was having little impact on those around me. We dug deeper, and I could see that any ministry role I was filling came, firstly, from a desire to know God for myself. I came across a Bible verse, Philippians 3:10-11, that I can genuinely identify with:

> [10]*I want to know Christ and experience the mighty power that raised him from the dead. I want to suffer with him, sharing in his death,* [11] *so that one way or another, I will experience the resurrection from the dead!*

The outcome of my sessions with a psychologist is that I value myself and take care of myself much more because I know much more about who I am and my purpose. Chatting with the psychologist enabled me to see the gap between my values and what I did. That gap is closing.

The chats help me to know why I respond in particular ways. I am so grateful for the eighteen months of (mostly) weekly visits because they also helped me enjoy my life while being more efficient and feeling more satisfied with work.

If you feel that you need to talk with a professional about your relationships and your emotional well-being, please take action. If one of your loved ones suggests that it would be good for you to talk to a psychologist, please listen and take action. If you've been through some significant traumas, get checked out for residual damage. It is worth the time and the money to be a better version of yourself.

As an interim step, you can visit websites like Get Your Headright: Digital Mental Health Solutions at http://getyourheadright.com.au/anxiety-and-depression-report and take the self-test. It is confidential, and you will get an email from a trained and qualified professional.

I'm very grateful for the professional help I've received. Having walked this journey until now, it is clear that we can develop emotional intelligence. I want to keep growing in this, to keep discovering more of who I am and why I respond in the ways that I do. You can also emerge healthier, more secure and more able to provide and care for those around you.

Jesus

I mentioned in the last chapter that one sign of burnout for me was the intensity of my prayer. I was very disciplined in prayer before burnout. I prayed for an hour every morning while walking around my pool. But as I approached burnout, there were no moments of peace or closeness to God. There was growing desperation. I only focused on problem-solving and strived to fill the gap of where I was versus where I wanted to be. My prayers focused on cultural aspects of success; money, numbers and statistics. They were prayers asking for quantity, not quality.

Once I began to feel replenished during my work leave, my prayer time took a very different approach. I sat in a comfortable chair. I started by being conscious of my breath and God's presence. I felt His presence filling my lungs. I focussed on affirming my relationship with Jesus and feeling His peace. I read some Bible passages, and then, finally, I pursued things in prayer where there needed to be a change or resolution. I prayed about the things and people on my heart. There is a place for pursuing solutions in prayer, but now, instead of letting problem-solving consume my prayers, I started with a sense of a secure attachment to God, one that is deep and life-giving.

When it comes to reading passages, I created a soundtrack of scriptures that would bring a sense of vitality to me. I formed a small list of Bible verses that spoke to me, to who I am and my identity rather than performance. The first verse was 1 John 3:1 (NLV) *"See what great love the Father has for us that He would call us His children. And that is what we are. For this reason, the people of the world do not know who we are because they did not know Him."* This verse has always been foundational to me, one I returned to when I wasn't feeling good about myself and disconnected from God and people. As I read that verse as a soundtrack to change what I was thinking in my head, I started to feel God's love for me.

The second verse was Ephesians 2:6 (NLV) *"God raised us up from death when He raised up Christ Jesus. He has given us a place with Christ in the heavens."* There were more verses to follow, all of which affirmed me and my relationship with God. I recited them over and over each morning. The principle behind this is that these verses helped change my thinking and shape my identity and perception to create the space and peace I needed to pray.

Family

Since Adrienne had her own journey in depression several years before my burnout, she could give great insight and knew that I would get through this difficult time. She knew that it was necessary to provide me with space to be well. I love the way she didn't make it personal. She never said that I wasn't giving her enough time or not pulling my weight. Adrienne was loving and thoughtful.

I know it was difficult for her because she was highly engaged in church leadership, as was my son, Josh, but neither brought difficulties or problems back to me. We were used to talking openly and often about the happenings at church. However, they both restrained from sharing too much, knowing that I needed the break from even thinking about work.

My children were also exceptional during this time. They didn't shield me from the personal things they were walking through, some of them quite difficult, but they didn't place an expectation on me to fix what I couldn't fix. I truly appreciated that we maintained family times to meet and eat together.

We had a family dinner in October, about six months into my work leave, when I was about to start back part-time. Adrienne, our three children and their partners all gathered and prayed with me. I felt so blessed that with the seeds I had sown, my children had become like strong trees with a faith in God that helped carry me through.

Psalm 127:3-5 (The Passion Translation)

³ Children are God's love-gift; they are heaven's generous reward.
⁴ Children born to a young couple will one day rise to protect
and provide for their parents.
⁵ Happy will be the couple who has many of them!
A household full of children will not bring shame on your name
but victory when you face your enemies,
for your offspring will have influence and honour
to prevail on your behalf!

Doctor: General Practitioner

I had seen my doctor over a long period of time—about 15 years before I entered burnout. He knew me and my history well. He was consistent and firm yet gentle and appropriate while handling my issues. When he strongly suggested I needed to take time off and I stubbornly assured him that was impossible, he didn't force it. He just said, "Well, I'll see you in a month." He knew that my difficulty was escalating. Looking back, I am so impressed with his insight and knowledge. This occurred still several years before burnout was classified as an occupational phenomenon.[28]

---

28 Burn-out an "occupational phenomenon": International Classification of Diseases. Word Health Organization. 28 May 2019. https://www.who.int/news/item/28-05-2019-burn-out-an-occupational-phenomenon-international-classification-of-diseases

In that first session, he suggested some counselling and gave me a mental health plan; ten sessions with a psychologist. It was a beneficial way to begin that journey.

On our second meeting, my blood test results were back, and he affirmed that there was nothing physically wrong with me. That, combined with the escalation of my symptoms, finally pushed me to trust what he was saying and take up his prescription: rest.

My GP had the conducting role for my health. He helped me get WorkCover, which required engaging with the State Government. He helped me get working insurance, which paid my wage at a hundred per cent for six months. Through that insurance, he also ensured that I had physiotherapy, psychological, and physical therapy and personally monitored me every few weeks during my most critical time.

If you feel that you might be burning out or know someone, it's imperative to have a medical professional assess you.

Back to Work

As I began to recover and feel more vital, the discussions began about returning to work. Initially, the doctor had prescribed three months off. That was reviewed monthly and extended to six months. It was decided that I could commence working part-time after consulting with my doctor, psychologist, WorkCover, and my team at work.

I took on 12 hours a week under the supervision of a back-to-work psychologist engaged by WorkCover—not the psychologist I met with personally. The back-to-work psychologist was there specifically to work with my team and me through the transition. They clarified what I could do and what I couldn't. A suitable duties programme was drawn up: I was to engage with a few team members I managed directly and could respond to work emails. I could do some general pastoring duties and visits. I was involved with service preparation and the weekly church service. I began chairing the monthly Board meetings. I was also guided to include replenishing activities, such as reading and further study. It was clear that I was not to take on crisis counselling appointments, like a couple with marriage problems, for instance. I was limited in using the work mobile and could answer calls only during work hours. Social media like Facebook was out, as were work emails where I was not on allocated work time.

Over the next twelve months, I slowly stepped up to full-time.

Several months into my return to work, I felt myself slipping backwards again. But was this just a feeling, or was it actually happening? Was I regressing? And how would I know if I was? Could I find something to measure how I was doing, like gauges on the car that alert us to what's going on? So, I started searching for measures of my health that I could easily see.

Reflection Questions for Chapter Three:

1. What are my replenishing activities?
2. Who will support me during recovery?
3. How would I rate my well-being in the following areas on a scale of 1 to 10?
    - Spirituality
    - Relationships
    - Emotional tank
    - General lifestyle/health
    - Areas of risk

CHAPTER FOUR

Creating Gauges

I felt good for nearly six months into my return to work. I was forming attachments, feeling productive and satisfied with my work and life. But then, I began to feel myself slipping. My insomnia was back, and I was battling anxiety and depression. I wanted to withdraw again. This time though, I felt more aware of my symptoms, things spinning out of control, and I needed to proceed with caution. From my burnout, I had developed some techniques and habits that I knew helped me with my symptoms, but I also knew what could be ahead of me. After all my hard work, I was frustrated that my actions hadn't been successful and depressed because I wasn't sure I could go through the entire process from the beginning.

I began to realise that this was something I might battle for the rest of my life. Burnout isn't a sickness like the flu that you catch from a virus and eventually get over; it comes from all the habits you have built into your lifestyle. Even after a rest, and some reflection and replenishment, you can't go back to the lifestyle you once had. In this regard, it's essential to understand what aspects of your lifestyle led you to burnout. I began to think about some safety measures I could set up so that things never got as bad as they did the first time.

Firstly, I looked at where my emotional tank was leaking. Was it spiritual? Financial? Emotional? Relational? Physical? I started making charts to gauge aspects of my life.

Over the years, I have heard a few people talk about the importance of reading your gauges, like having a dashboard of a car—gauges that indicate how you are travelling, show the sustainability of the trip and serve to help you make the journey safely. Car gauges have warning lights indicating things like low oil, low fuel, imminent threats to the safety of the vehicle and occupants. If I could track my symptoms, I could know when I was approaching danger. If I could chart how I react to different elements of my life, I could understand what led me to feel these symptoms and then avoid them. I could understand what replenished me. I could take the time to partake in these activities when I felt depleted.

Burnout Gauge: Physical Symptoms of Emotional Depletion

I began by looking at ways to measure my emotional well-being, but it can be difficult to measure feelings. Perhaps, I could rate my daily emotions on some kind of scale? But was there a better way to get a picture of my health? I wanted to find something more empirical and verifiable. Therefore, I began to look for indicators of emotional depletion for myself. I looked for measurable, physical symptoms that I knew were related to my emotional state.

Eventually, I found three strong indicators, and I started charting them each week: insomnia, heart palpitations, and fatigue.

For me, insomnia is always one of the earliest signs of stress. I began to ask how many nights this week have I had trouble sleeping? My pattern of insomnia tended to be either having difficulty going to sleep or going to sleep but then waking during the night and laying awake for an hour or so. Things were churning in my emotions, keeping me from sleeping. I realised that I hadn't slept well for the past three nights that week. I remembered that in February of the previous year, I was having trouble about four nights a week, yet a couple of months before, I had been sleeping well. Seeing the three nights for the week listed on the chart was a clear danger sign.

On one of those nights, I noticed that my heart was pounding. Even though I had not gotten up, I was aware that my heart was rapid and strong. My professionals called these rapid or irregular heartbeats palpitations. In this case, there was no physical cause like exertion or sickness. So, I added palpitations to my chart as another warning sign.

Years ago, I wanted to build a wine cellar in our new house, as wines don't keep well in our subtropical climate. However, we decided to purchase a second-hand wine fridge instead due to financial priorities. I researched a fridge of good quality and found a Vintec on sale locally. It worked well at the seller's home, but unbeknown to me, I damaged it in transit. When I turned it on, it ran and ran but did not come down to the temperature I had selected. I could smell the motor getting hot, and the wines were not cooling. So, I turned it off and found a repair person who replaced the damaged copper pipe and re-gassed the fridge. The motor now runs until the set temperature is reached, then shuts off until it needs to cool again. I was like a fridge motor low on gas. When a fridge is low on gas, it continues to run, but the motor will just burn out if the gas is not replenished. When I am not exerting physical energy, my rapid heart rate signals high stress and my emotional tank is low. My charts soon revealed that palpitations mainly occurred when I was also battling insomnia.

Not only was I having palpitations and difficulty sleeping, but I also started to feel the symptoms of fatigue again; chronic tiredness, dizziness, aching muscles, muscle and joint weakness, slow responses, impaired decision-making, and irritability. As I reflected on this, I could see there was only one day that week I was not fatigued. My head was clear, sharp, decisive that day. I was full of energy, strong in joints and muscles.

While it was confronting to chart and note these indicators, I was pleased to have things I could tangibly verify. My emotions were all over the place, and my mind was foggy, but these had an actuality—they were observable. I could do more than guess how I was; I now had three markers that indicated my emotional well-being. Consequently, it became clear that I was in trouble once more and needed to address this or I would crash again.

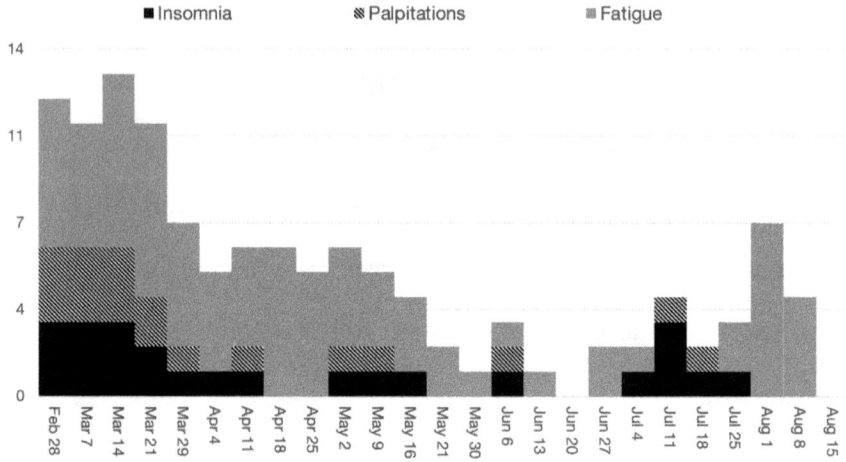

Burnout Symptoms Chart

Here, I chart and observe physical measures of emotional depletion. The most important thing is the observation, which helped me see what I was not seeing, and consequently, become more self-aware and alerted me to grave danger in my emotional health. It's like keeping a logbook of the journey.

For many years, we had an 835i BMW, a graceful and majestic old girl. One day, while Adrienne was driving, the oil light came on. The car stopped at the next set of traffic lights, and people came running up to the car, shouting that the car was on fire, calling Adrienne out and turning off the motor. The autopsy showed that the gearbox gasket had sprung a leak. The highly flammable gearbox oil had then spilled onto the hot muffler, caught alight, and thick black smoke billowed from beneath the car. Fortunately, when the car stopped, the pressure on the oil in the gearbox lowered, the oil stopped feeding the fire, and the fire had burnt out by the time the fire brigade arrived. My dear Adrienne was safe, but our mechanic pronounced the car terminal.

The oil, temperature gauge, and brake lights all indicate serious problems, each having the potential to stop the journey. When they show together, serious mechanical attention is imperative. Emotional depletion stresses our body like low oil and high temperature in a vehicle. When all the warning lights are on, it means it's time to stop now and get help. If insomnia, palpitations or chronic fatigue are showing, it likewise means *stop and get help!*

I could have also charted detachment and work satisfaction. Coupled with emotional depletion, these are the three significant components of burnout. The aim of these charts is to build self-awareness.

For detachment, I observed my activity on my iPhone during time with another person. I noticed that just like last time, as my detachment from people increased, I became addicted to my smartphone and iPad. Although I didn't chart this, I asked myself, "Am I on my phone when with other people, thereby deflecting or avoiding the connections?"

I try to reflect on my conversations about people constantly. If I find myself getting cynical and critical of others, I know I'm becoming depleted, and it's time for me to fill up. Also, I observe my attention to people in face-to-face conversations. Sometimes, I find myself looking past them at other people, which signals both to them and me that I am not connecting in the conversation. I say to myself in those moments, "Settle and listen."

For work satisfaction, I focus on things I am responsible for rather than what I can't change. I am not responsible for how people respond, but I am responsible for delivering the message in the best way I can so they can hear and understand me well. I pull away from things that make me compare myself to others, for example limiting my time on Instagram. After delivering a message, I ask listeners questions like, "How did this help you?" I seek affirmation rather than believe it's more noble to deny myself of others' praise.

While my emotional health was improving, my emotions seemed to gain more colour—I was increasingly allowing myself to feel. I was becoming more conscious of my emotions. But as I felt myself slipping backward, I also experienced my emotions become duller.

These were the major indicators that showed me I was heading back to serious trouble. I highly recommend anyone facing burnout create their own list of indicators and chart them. Others may need to monitor different things, as stress affects us differently. Be aware of your danger signs and how often you are experiencing them.

Gauge: Overall Well-Being

After taking the time to track my emotional depletion, I had the evidence that I was in decline. I needed to look at getting healthy again, and therefore, I decided to gauge my overall health in the most significant areas of my life. I listed areas that I could easily quantify; spiritual, financial, emotional, relational and physical. To obtain overall measures, I added a median average, which takes out the highs and lows. I began charting this based on a gut-level response.

Here is my chart from February 18th through May 16th, rating areas in my life from zero to ten—zero being "I can't get out of bed" to ten "I'm doing great." And then, for good measure, or more accurately, to give me a snapshot, I added a graph that tracked the median.

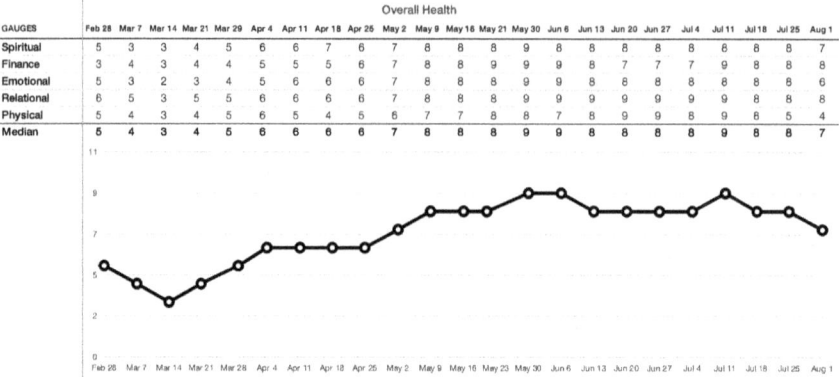

As I reflected on my chart over the first couple of weeks, I started asking the question, "Why am I feeling emotionally lower?" I realised I was in grief. I was preparing to say goodbye to a role I had for ten years–that of National Operations Manager of C3 Church. A large part of my identity was wrapped in this role. I also knew this would impact relationships, that the time spent together with people who had become quite close friends would significantly diminish. The unsolved financial stress of not having the role compounded the grief. No wonder I was not sleeping, my heart racing and my body feeling fatigued again.

Yet, I knew from the journey so far that recovery was not only possible but achievable.

Buoyancy Gauge

My desire for well-being and vitality made me want to quantify the things that fill my tank, as well as the negative symptoms I was experiencing. I wanted to understand what was really making a difference in my emotional well-being and, even more than that, when the drain on the tank is too large to compensate by intentionally increasing the activities that build emotional vitality.

I learned that it was mainly up to me to pay attention to my emotional tank's level. Being on this journey for eleven months at this stage, I knew many of the activities that replenished me, for example, regular exercise, three times a week at least, helped me feel good. The release of endorphins during exercise made me happy. I continued to see my psychologist since it positively affected how I viewed myself.

My replenishing recreational activities ranged from creating something from wood to hanging out with my grandchildren, to breakfast with some mates. I also added two very simple things: walking and breathing. Simple as they are, they do make a profound difference. I love taking a vigorous walk: half an hour at a speed that makes it difficult to carry on a conversation helps me the most.

Breathing has been an incredible tool: breathing in while counting in ten (if possible) and out, counting to ten—big, full-belly breaths. I try to practise breathing slowly when I wake and when I'm going to sleep. Sometimes, that means I go back to sleep in the morning. And usually, when I'm going to sleep, I do so very quickly. Sometimes, during the day, I'll lie down in a hammock or on my bed, and after slowly breathing for a while, I'll end up drifting off. I wake feeling refreshed. As a result of learning to value myself, I now find it easy to permit myself to replenish.

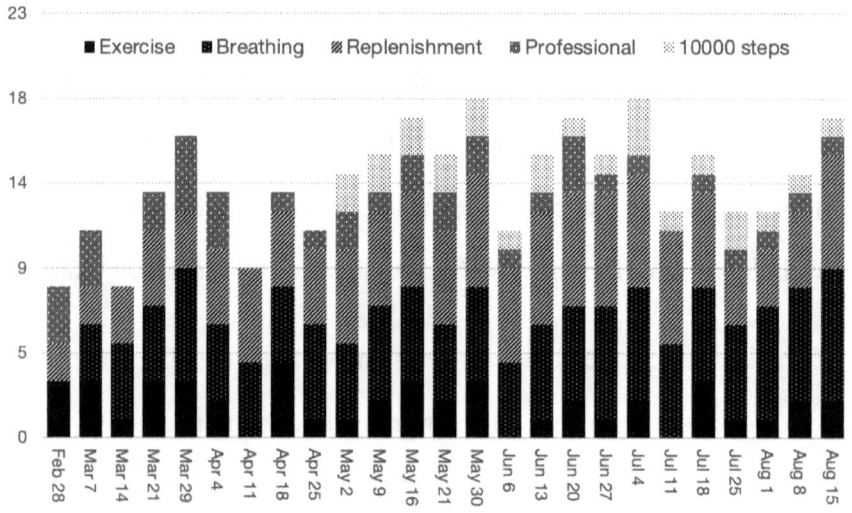

One of the questions I ask myself when I'm completing my weekly emotional health review is, "What do I need to build into my coming week to compensate for the depletion of last week?" I do this at the beginning of my week as I adjust my calendar looking ahead. As the pace increases, I build increased buoyancy activities into my routine. Twelve months after the professional help had finished, I re-engaged with my psychologist and my exercise physiologist. I asked them to help me, as mentors, to keep watch over me and help me further develop my mental and physical health.

What Depletes Me

I started reflecting on the activities, events, or situations that consistently depleted my emotional tank, or caused me to detach from people or gave me significant dissatisfaction with work and life. It took me over six months, but after a lot of thought on this matter, I found that eight things have the potential to push me toward burnout.

Initially, I listed the obvious adverse events of life: Conflict, overwork, dilemmas and broken relationships. These seemed to be universally negative and always lead to stress. When I started back at work, I was able to add two more unexpected depletions to my list: management and preaching. It was surprising because both areas have always been strengths of mine, and I had previously found them stimulating. It frustrated me. I finally added sickness and psychological stress.

Some of these areas are specific to me and my life. Your list of gauges could look very different. For instance, you may become stressed by large social gatherings. Perhaps your boss is challenging to deal with. You may have a family member you love dearly but often puts you in difficult situations. Your gauges will not be the same as mine. It's essential to take the time to reflect on your own life, to measure the areas that constantly leave you feeling drained.

Here, I'll break down why each of these negative impacts became an important gauge for my mental health:

Conflict: Few people find that conflict charges them. If you are, you probably shouldn't be in an enterprise that helps people flourish. Conflict seems to stem from anger and frustration between two or more people but actually stems from feelings of hurt or being dismissed. Conflict can come out of an intense situation, causing people to react strongly immediately. Still, more often than not, conflict begins without us realising, with tension building subtly until there is a breaking point. In Australia, we often refer to this breaking point as a "kick in the gut." When that happens, the force of impact causes an involuntary exhale of air and muscle spasms, leaving one breathless and gasping for air. This can also be how it feels emotionally.

Conflict can have a positive outcome. It can bring understanding, clarity and eventually, working in harmony. As Hart says in his book *Safe Haven Marriage*; "Conflict is often a way you and your spouse discover the truth about each other and come to terms with your differences."[29] It is part of good relationships. However, it requires emotional energy. Even well-managed conflict will take its toll on your emotional tank.

Overwork: Overworking has been a clear theme in my writing so far. Just to restate a definition: overworking is working beyond your capacity. The success-oriented, high-achieving, make-it-happen people are more prone to burnout. But overwork is not just in the temperaments of certain people: it has become part of the fabric of our society. Our culture promotes success and the idea that the destination, more than the journey, is all that matters— reaching a certain status, an amount of money, a size of house or a type of car. We value each other by our things and our accomplishments.

Dilemmas: A dilemma requires a choice between two or more alternative situations. Sometimes, all possibilities seem satisfactory, sometimes unsatisfactory, or a combination of these.

Broken Relationships: Hurt and detachment in relationships can be one of the most significant triggers for depletion. Nothing quite affects our hearts like our relationships, and because people can be complicated and messy, they are often the most difficult stressors to

---

[29]Hart, Archibald; Morris, Sharon. Safe Haven Marriage (p. 61). Thomas Nelson. Kindle Edition.

avoid. We bleed in the place where a relationship is broken.

Queensland has some beautiful rainforest walks. They are somewhat magical when humidity is high, and it's raining. After one such walk during a romantic stay at a rainforest cottage, I discovered leeches had attached to my legs. I quickly removed these slippery, slimy things. There was not much pain as they came off, but I did begin to bleed. Leeches inject hirudin, an anticoagulant, into the blood, causing it to flow out from the wound. Like hirudin, broken relationships cause us to bleed and keep on bleeding.

We don't always think about how the effects of broken relationships spread if they go unaddressed. Children suffer from their parents' divorce. A wife suffers from her husband's broken relationship with his parents. When dealing with pain in their relationships, even our friends can pass the effects onto us. Scars from past relationships almost always resurface somehow unless we take the time to understand our pain and use it to grow into healthier people.

Managing people: I have always liked working with others. I love being involved in a community. I love helping others solve problems and leading those in need. I've always considered myself to be good at managing my team. However, working with other people naturally leads to conflict, dilemmas, and more complex organisational issues. It requires thinking about the big picture and balancing many needs. After returning to work from my leave, I found it so much more exhausting than I once did. I still enjoy it, but it takes a more considerable toll than before.

Preaching: I love preaching and find great satisfaction in delivering what I hear God saying to people, but I added it to the list as I realised my tank needed filling after pouring out my heart through preaching. Even Jesus experienced depletion in pursuing his mission. When a woman desiring healing reached out and touched him, he said, "Someone touched me; I know that power has gone out from me."[30] Not only what we regard as adverse events of life can be depleting, but also the things we treasure and love.

Physical Sickness: Sickness is somewhat obvious but important to note as a depleting thing. When we are sick, the world is greyer, life is tougher, and challenges are bigger, in addition to the toll it takes on our physical health. We often forget how connected our physical, mental and emotional health are—sickness in one area will eventually affect the others. We must tend to them all and tread carefully when feeling depleted in any aspect.

---

[30] Luke 8:46 (NIV)

Psychological stress: This is an encompassing term for a negative relationship with your environment, particularly overwhelming situations that evoke a strong emotional and physiological reaction. These, for me, are things like moving house, abuse, manipulation, and the death of a loved one (including a loved pet).

It can be something subtle, like a quietly incessant, irritating, dripping tap, or it can be painful and obvious, like a large splinter in a finger that just festers away. This stress may be a broken relationship or finding yourself trapped in debt and unable to find work. It could be knowing something about someone and not being able to share it.

You are probably wondering why I didn't include grief—that is because the major trigger for grief is a broken relationship, whether the loss of a family member, friend or a person who breaks connection.

Most of these are very easy to measure and quickly see if they occur. My analytical mind led to keeping a weekly bar-stacking chart because I wanted to see the cumulative effect. When I see the chart stacking to over 3 in a week, my emotional tank has gone from one draining point to multiple. Then I know that I need to pay extra attention to my well-being by spending extra time on replenishment activities.

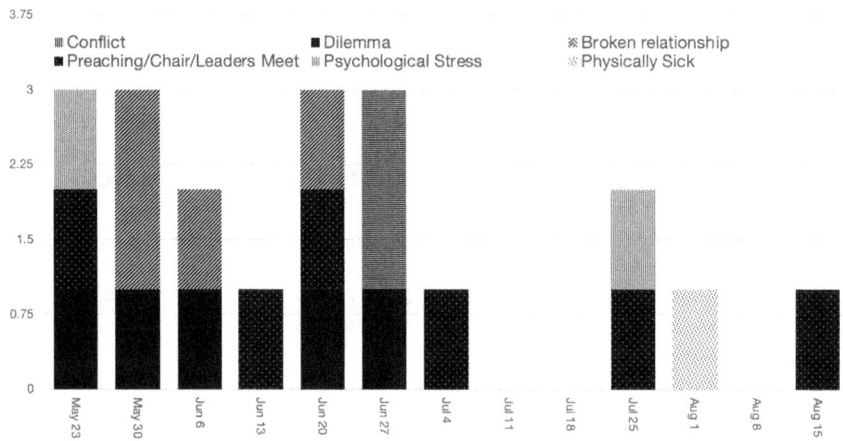

Results

So, in the end, what came from all this work? All these measurements and charts? All the time I spent reflecting and gauging the effects?

As I tracked my physical symptoms, my replenishing activities and the activities that depleted me over the months, you can see I began to get better. I had fewer symptoms as I became more self-aware. Monitoring them has been helpful as it shows me when I need to increase buoyancy activities and minimise depleters where possible. The worse my symptoms, the more I would focus on logging replenishing activities instead of depleting ones. It took time, but I eventually began to feel more in control.

What I did was create a system to build my self-awareness. Even though I had grown more and more aware of the things that deplete and replenish me, I found it valuable to track them because this led to so many new insights.

For many, burnout never entirely goes away. You may improve and feel different, but burnout will keep returning unless you take care of yourself the way you need to. At its core, the solution to burnout is self-value and self-care.

Depleters have a cumulative effect. My burnout was caused by sustained stress over a long time. I have discovered that when my chart shows three depleters, it's not just $1+1+1=3$, but more like $3^2=9$. The cumulative stress is greater than the sum of the individual stresses. So, I know I need to be careful when they mount up. I encourage you to understand what depletes you, especially if you are slipping into unhealthy habits. The principle here is to discover your threshold and what is sustainable for you.

Make a list and review it over several months. Track your results and adjust your lifestyle as needed. Without your mental, emotional and physical health, you aren't entirely you, and you can't offer all of the wonderful aspects of yourself to others. Take care of yourself and value yourself as much as the people around you do.

Here's How to Get Started.

Know your symptoms.

List your most significant signs of stress and begin to track them. How often do they happen to you? Every day or every few days? Rate them on a scale of 1 to 10, depending on how severely they affect you.

Identify your depleters and monitor them.

Once you know the symptoms, begin to note when they occur. Are there any consistencies? Do they happen in the morning? At night? Following certain activities? Once you see connections to potential stressors in your life, begin to chart these as well.

Know what replenishes you.

As you start to see correlations between your symptoms and your stressors, it's time to make some changes. If you can take specific stressors out of your routine, do it! What is one thing that stresses you that you could change? However, there will be unavoidable stressors. Try following these draining activities with replenishing ones. If you had a difficult day at work, plan for a quiet night and an early bedtime. After conflict with your spouse, plan a relaxing and fun activity you enjoy together.

Find someone to help you.

I am grateful for my mentor who helped me build awareness of depleters through his feedback. He also helped me take ownership of change, for example, helping me identify what steps I could take to repair broken relationships.

Weekly Review.

Take time to review these weekly. Add anything else that you notice to the charts. I am confident that the buoyancy measures work for all. But depleters will be different for different people.

Reflection Questions for Chapter Four:

1) What are some tangible and empirical signs that I'm stressed?
2) How is my overall well-being?

    - spiritually

    - financially

    - emotionally

    - relationally

    - physically

3) In what ways do I replenish myself, and how often am I engaging in them?
4) What depletes me, and how often do these activities/events occur?
5) Who can help me identify stress and minimise it?

CHAPTER FIVE

Preventing Burnout

What can I do to prevent burnout?

People frequently ask what I could have done to prevent burnout from happening in the first place. How could I have prepared and protected myself? What differences could I have made in my life so this wouldn't have happened? Of course, there are a few easy answers; remove some pressure from life, don't push so hard, make more time to rest. In hindsight, these are all obvious solutions, but all of these things are easier said than done. High-achieving and driven people rarely make time for rest and replenishment. Generally, it won't occur to people like me to ease up before it's too late.

More valuable and reasonable is to work two things into your life: self-awareness and time with mentors. These things will help you see your life in the bigger picture and balance the areas you value. I think that if I had spent more time listening to the voices around me and paying attention to what my body and heart were telling me, I could have avoided a lot of pain.

Self-awareness

Despite what you may have been taught, self-awareness is something you can practise and build by making time for reflection—paying attention to the internal reactions and feelings you experience in different situations. There is a lot about ourselves left to discover. Do you ever feel riled into sudden anger and can't quite lay your finger on why? Do you occasionally feel depressed, though nothing seems particularly different about your day? Do you find yourself agreeing to things you don't want to do? There are so many ways we behave and feel throughout our day, usually without considering why. However, the more we are aware of the whys, the more we can control how we feel and behave. Understanding our feelings allows us to act appropriately and know what we need.

According to Chris Adams of Azusa Pacific University and Matt Bloom of University of Notre Dame, "self-awareness will actually develop our resilience; by 'resilience,' we mean a person's capacity to respond to the changing and sometimes challenging world around them."[31] They suggest that there are three dimensions of resilience: self-awareness, self-reflectivity, and self-control. Self-awareness leads to self-reflectivity, which is "the ability to examine and think about our thoughts, feelings and behaviours, especially in terms of whether or not they are appropriate, good, helpful, or otherwise positive for ourselves, other people, and the world around us."[32] Self- reflectivity then allows us to build the capacity for self-control, that is, "to change things in ourselves and the world around us. It also comprises our ability to set and achieve goals in life."[33] Together, self-awareness, self-reflectivity and self-control will help set boundaries in your life, prioritise what matters and understand yourself to a greater degree. When life does become challenging (there will always be those moments), practising these three competencies will lead you to have greater resilience.

Mentors

I want to emphasise, again, how important mentors are in the prevention of and recovery from burnout. Even the most self-aware person will have some blind spots. No matter how much we practise

---

31 Adams, Bloom 2017

32 Adams, Bloom 2017

33 Adams, Bloom 2017

self-reflectivity and self-control, there are just some things that we cannot see in ourselves. In the same way that we can't see the skyline of a city while we're in the centre of it, we can't always see the entire picture of ourselves. Finding a mentor is key to helping us see the big picture for self-care and burnout prevention.

Note that a mentoring role is very different from a coaching role. As a person who has spent a lot of time coaching and being coached, I want to make this distinction: a coaching role, to put it simply, is about what to do and how you are doing it, aiming to help you perform better in a specific area. Coaching is important, and indeed, people do better through coaching. Mentoring, however, is more all-encompassing, with the primary goal being personal development.

Finding a mentor to help you through the challenging times in your life and any time of life is a great way to gain a broader perspective. Find someone who asks intelligent questions and can respond without bias or judgement to your situation, who knows you and can see you regularly yet isn't too involved in the daily aspects of your personal life. A mentor can say things that close friends and family members often can't. Sometimes, we respond to their observations better because we know they are more impartial than the deeply entwined people in our lives. Mentors should have more life experience and wisdom and should be people we can rely on to provide truthful insights and advice. For mentors to be a good resource, we must come to them with honesty and openness, willing to trust them with our vulnerabilities.

But how do you find a great mentor? I have the belief that if you seek, you find. My encouragement is to start looking. Mentors can form naturally in your life, but if you don't feel you have one, this is an opportunity to ask someone you respect and admire for some help. Some professionals mentor for a living. I met my mentor, Keith Farmer, at a National Director's meeting I was organising. He was giving a session on the importance of sabbatical and rest. I went to him afterwards and asked for him to both mentor me and teach me to mentor others. He has worked with me, asking caring and perceptive questions to help me build self-awareness.

Pastors, the key factor for a safe mentoring relationship is to have a mentor outside of your chain of command, whether in your movement or denomination or a different stream altogether.

What are the competencies of a good mentor? Good mentors themselves need to be healthy to recognise the signs of emotional depletion in the people around them. They need to be able to talk honestly about what they see. A mentor has three significant abilities; discernment, feedback, and inspiring change by helping you imagine a healthy future.

The amount of time you should spend with your mentor will vary based on your situation. For some, it's about sustaining health and preventing burnout. In this case, a quarterly check-in is all that is needed to make a positive change in your life. But if you need to be lifted out of burnout, monthly or even weekly is likely necessary.

If you are having trouble finding a mentor in your own life, the team VerveLead could help.

Reducing Vocational Risks

While ultimately, the responsibility for the care of our mental, physical and emotional health falls on ourselves, there are so many ways that workplaces can eliminate or reduce burnout. A healthy work environment makes a huge difference; the team will be happier, more productive and efficient, and the turn-over rates will remain low—it benefits everyone. The responsibility falls on Board members, managers and employers to create a healthy work environment.

Employers/Boards

The role of the Board in dealing with and assisting burnout prevention is paramount. I am very grateful for the stellar way the C3 Robina Board operated during my burnout, adopting a caretaker role and carefully managing the church during my absence. With assistance from our church overseer, I appointed an acting chairperson and an acting senior minister. Together with the Board members, these endeavoured to keep true to the church's vision and watch over its safety while attending to the corporate legal and fiduciary responsibilities. Even though income was reduced during my absence, the church's financial bottom line improved. Expenditure was meticulously monitored and, when possible, reduced. The Board endorsed the application to WorkCover for a claim, which when approved meant financial pressure was relieved.

One of the contributing factors to my initial burnout was that I did not disclose to the Board my emotional well-being. They knew I was working hard, but I thought it was not the place to express weakness or difficulty trying to be the leader. Never in a Board meeting did I say, "I have too much work to do", or "This incident we are dealing with has seriously affected me emotionally", or "I am suffering great grief over the loss of these people", or "My tank is empty." In retrospect, I wish I had shared how certain situations and dilemmas felt very uncomfortable and dangerous for me. Doing so would have helped me feel understood and possibly encouraged others around me to feel more comfortable sharing their feelings.

If the key leader is not doing well, the organisation will suffer. After my leave of absence began, the Board added "Senior Ministers' Health" to the agenda to normalise talking about our mental and emotional health and create a safe space to ask for what we need. Questions like, "Is your workload reasonable?", "How well are we providing for your financial needs?" and "What part of your workload is energy-producing and life-giving?" Everything rises and falls on leadership. If the key leader is not doing well, the organisation will suffer. Therefore, it's in the Board's best interest to do what they can to help their employees thrive.

A healthy workplace requires an atmosphere of trust, a collegiate mentality, where together we are working to accomplish the organisation's vision. This takes time and effort from all. Sometimes, pessimism and negativity, often influenced by each person's circumstances in life, can creep into a Board. A handbrake mentality of opposition and correction will never achieve a safe workplace environment. Therefore, make changes to the team when necessary, primarily fighting for a healthy team.

I am grateful that my team did not try to shoot me when I was sick but sought to bandage my wounds and give space for my healing. If WorkCover had not been available, we would have been in severe difficulty. We had Key Person insurance but only in the event of death. In hindsight, we also should have had wage cover and disability insurance. So, please look at your insurances and take necessary action to see that you are covered.

As chair of your Boards, senior ministers, please never complain about the men and women God has given you. Take courage, be the leader and take them where God calls you to go. We are agents of change: our Board is what we make it.

To members of the Board, thank you for your willingness to serve God and his church in this way. Work with, believe the best, communicate, stay fresh in God because building a church is a spiritual contest. Schools, corporations and governance also have Boards, but in the church, the vital need for spirituality (one of the five core competencies) and the enterprise of bringing light into places of darkness can wear you down. There is an added layer of pressure to do good and be excellent in everything you do.

I encourage you to give this book to your Board members. "The health of your leader will determine the health of your church"[34]. One of your responsibilities is to protect the assets of your entity or church. In

---

34 quote Bill Hybels, Courageous Leadership

Christian terms, this understanding is found in passages like Ephesians 4:11 which describes people as Christ's gifts to the church:

> *Now these are the gifts Christ gave to the church: the apostles, the prophets, the evangelists, and the pastors and teachers.*

Emma Seppala from Stanford University says "the data is clear: engagement is key, it's what we should strive for as leaders and employees. But what we want is smart engagement—the kind that leads to enthusiasm, motivation and productivity, without the burnout. Increased demands on employees need to be balanced with increased resources—particularly before important deadlines and during other times of stress."[35]

It is advised that Boards prepare and implement a strategy for the well-being of their key employees. SafeWork Australia and WorkSafe NZ outline the obligation of Boards to care for the physiological health of their employees: that is to prevent harm, intervene early and support recovery. Authorising funding for mentoring is a great step in this responsibility because it monitors health and builds sustainable well-being. Also, because workers have a duty of care for their own health and safety, it is most reasonable for a key employee to request funding

---

35 https://hbr.org/2018/02/1-in-5-highly-engaged-employees-is-at-risk-of-burnout

for mentoring from their Board. [36]

The Australian Catholic University's study on School Principals in Australia recommends that employers make the following choices to reduce and prevent burnout in their employees:

1. *Take the moral choice* of reducing job demands or increasing job resources to allow school leaders to cope with the increased demands. Better still, do both. This will help to increase the level of social capital in schools.

2. *Trust rather than rule educators.* Leave the mechanisms for producing the best educators to the experienced educators themselves. This will also increase social capital. Long-term increases in social capital helped Finland become the world leader in education.[37]

---

36 "Mental Health." *Safe Work Australia*, 7 June 2018, www.safeworkaustralia.gov.au/topic/mental-health.

"Work-Related Psychological Health and Safety: A Systematic Approach to Meeting Your Duties." *Safe Work Australia*, 21 Jan. 2019, www.safeworkaustralia.gov.au/doc/work-related-psychological-health-and-safety-systematic-approach-meeting-your-duties.

37 Riley, P., See, S-M., Marsh, H. & Dicke, T. (2020) The Australian Principal Occupational Health, Safety and well-being Survey (IPPE Report). Sydney: Institute for PositivePsychology and Education, Australian Catholic University. Pg 6.

Taking care of Key Leaders

When considering the work of your staff, it's essential to know that executives carry greater loads than most of your employees. They run a greater risk of burnout—they often work under higher pressure, have more significant crises and dilemmas under their responsibility, and often deal with sustained stress over the years. The wellness of your executives, managers and other leaders in your team will also affect their employees. A healthy executive can better provide good leadership, see what their team needs, handle conflict and implement solutions.

School leaders are one example. A 2019 study of Australian Principals by the Australian Catholic University Institution for Positive Psychology and Education shares that, "School leaders continue to report sheer quantity of work, lack of time to focus on teaching and learning, and student mental health, as their main sources of stress. Mental health of students and staff has become an increasing source of stress for participants in recent years, with it being highest in 2019."[38]

Additionally, the ACU's study describes stressors experienced by a

---

[38] Riley, P., See, S-M., Marsh, H. & Dicke, T. (2020) The Australian Principal Occupational Health, Safety and well-being Survey (IPPE Report). Sydney: Institute for PositivePsychology and Education, Australian Catholic University. Pg 6.

school leader: "Over 84% of school leaders reported being subjected to offensive behaviour over the last year, with 51% reported having received threats of violence, and over 42% being exposed to physical violence. Compared to the general population, school leaders reported huge effect size higher for emotional demands, demands for hiding emotions, and work-family conflict. For health and well-being subscales, school leaders reported very large effect sizes for burnout, sleeping troubles and stress compared to the general population."[39]

Placing value on good mental health for your executives will show a value for mental health in everyone, allowing for more honest conversations, better self-care and a better all-around environment in which to work. Burnout is contagious. When one person pushes themself past their limit, it creates expectations of others to do the same. Once operating on adrenaline, they are more prone to avoidance or conflict, thereby negatively affecting the overall environment and adding to the stress of others around them. It is the job of leaders to set an example of self-care and encourage others to do the same.

The same study from 2009, gives some strategies for improving the well-being of school leaders, starting with professional support; "in

---

[39] Riley, P., See, S-M., Marsh, H. & Dicke, T. (2020) *The Australian Principal Occupational Health, Safety and well-being Survey* (IPPE Report). Sydney: Institute for PositivePsychology and Education, Australian Catholic University. Pg 6.

other emotionally demanding professions, such as psychology and social work, high levels of professional support and debriefing are standard procedures. This is not so in education. As a result, the average school leaders' well-being is less optimal than the average citizen. The school leaders who identified as coping least well with their daily tasks had the lowest levels of professional support from colleagues and superiors, while those who coped the best, reported the highest levels of professional support." [40]

When creating strategies for well-being for your employees, firstly assess which behaviours you are celebrating and rewarding? If you are celebrating and rewarding those who achieve at their own emotional risk, you are creating unhealthy standards. It may feel counterintuitive to allow time off and to encourage work-life boundaries because you fear less will get done, but a healthy team will be even more productive and produce better work than a team struggling with anxiety and stress. If you are interested in reading more about providing or getting professional support, finding or becoming a mentor, information and strategies are abundant on Verve Lead's website.[41]

---

[40] Riley, P., See, S-M., Marsh, H. & Dicke, T. (2020) The Australian Principal Occupational Health, Safety and well-being Survey (IPPE Report). Sydney: Institute for PositivePsychology and Education, Australian Catholic University. Pg 11.

[41] https://vervelead.com

Ministry and Care-Giving Professions: At Risk Vocations

Particular vocations are at higher risk for burnout. For instance, caregiving professionals are more likely to fall prey to overwork, anxiety and running on adrenaline. I want to focus this section on burnout within one of those caregiving professions—the ministry.

In their article, "Flourishing in Ministry: Well-being at Work in Helping Professions", Matt Bloom and Chris Adams write, "Those involved in helping professions often confront the worst kinds of evil as they work to help victims of violence, natural disaster, and economic deprivation. They may work in difficult and under-resourced settings. They may work in dangerous contexts where they are subject to violence and disasters themselves. In addition, the work itself is hard, complex, and seems to be never-ending. They act on faith that, somehow, good will come from all of their efforts. So workdays often unfold one after another without reward, rest or respite. Doing this kind of work well often requires denying one's own needs as one strives to serve others. This necessary self-denial—what we call positive sacrifice—is part of the experience of thriving, in part because it confirms that we are giving our best to something profoundly important. However, our research suggests that pastors and other caring professionals can tip from positive sacrifice into negative sacrifice (experiences that erode well-being) without realising they have made this transition. Negative sacrifice looks and feels like its positive cousin but is, in fact, a condition in which a person is experiencing too much fatigue, too much stress, and too many resource expenditures. We think that over time, negative sacrifice can lead to a host of problems, most notably burnout."[42]

Clergy, pastors, ordained ministers of the gospel, reverends, lead ministers, or whatever they labelled, people in these vocations are prone to burnout. The complexity of their work and their Christian convictions make them unique.

In another article, "A Burden Too Heavy",[43] Matt Bloom cites Richard Deshon, Professor at Michigan State university. "Dr. Richard Deshon is one of the leading experts on job analysis, a sophisticated research methodology for systematically determining the tasks, activities, and responsibilities of a particular job."[44] Deshon says, "The breadth of tasks performed by local church pastors coupled with the rapid switching between task clusters and roles that appears prevalent

---

42 Chris Adams, Matt Bloom, Journal of Psychology and Christianity 2017, Vol. 36, No. 3, 258

43 Dr Matt Bloom https://workwellresearch.com/media/images/FIM%20Report%20Workload.pdf

44 Dr Matt Bloom https://workwellresearch.com/media/images/FIM%20Report%20Workload.pdf

in this position is unique. I have never encountered such a fast-paced job with such varied and impactful responsibilities." [45]

Dr Deshon worked with the United Methodist Church to identify thirteen major task clusters that comprise the role of pastor. Each cluster comprises a wide variety of activities including administration, caregiving, facility-management and construction, preaching and public worship, evangelism, and communication. Dr Deshon also determined that in order to perform all of these tasks effectively, it would require sixty-four different personal competencies. He concluded that "it is almost inconceivable to imagine that a single person could be uniformly high on the sixty-four distinct knowledge, skills, abilities, and personal characteristics."[46] So a leading expert in job analysis concluded that it takes sixty-four competencies and that it's inconceivable for a person to have all these!

It's important to note that this study was carried out in Methodist churches in the USA, which is centrally managed and has centrally-owned property. Independent churches, which by nature have their own legal entities, require another set of competencies. Here, lead ministers need to also be legally savvy, fiduciarily responsible, comply

---

[45] Dr Matt Bloom https://workwellresearch.com/media/images/FIM%20Report%20Workload.pdf p1

[46] Dr Matt Bloom https://workwellresearch.com/media/images/FIM%20Report%20Workload.pdf

with corporate expectations, and possess some knowledge in property acquisition and development—that is, to have competencies in law, accounting, financial management, negotiation, architecture and interior design, traffic flow, acoustic impact, wildlife impact, arborist skills, and be able to relate to local councillors. And, if you live in Queensland as we do, be able to deal with snakes. Our church has a lot of children on site, both before and after school, and during school holidays. We have had a two-meter king brown snake sunning itself on the path on a few occasions. They are highly poisonous, and Queensland has the highest casualty rate in Australia.[47]

Bible teacher and author, Tony Cooke, jokes that the job description for a Senior Pastor sometimes feels like it demands a person is "able to leap tall buildings in a single bound, be more powerful than a locomotive, faster than a speeding bullet, walk on water, give policies to God.[48] It has been said that even the Apostle Paul would not qualify for a senior pastor job today! But levity aside, studies have shown that clergy are more prone to physical difficulties than their local constituents. The Duke Clergy Health Initiative[49] reports, "A study of

---

47 https://en.wikipedia.org/wiki/List_of_fatal_snake_bites_in_Australia

48 http://www.tonycooke.org/stories-and-illustrations/job_description/

49 https://divinity.duke.edu/initiatives/clergy-health-initiative

95% of the United Methodist clergy in North Carolina found that the clergy had higher rates of obesity, diabetes, arthritis and hypertension than other North Carolinians, even after demographic adjustments."[50] The clergy obesity rate was a startling 11 percentage points higher (40% versus 29%).

Although studies on the physical health of clergy are few, high rates of obesity among Lutheran pastors have also been found (Halaas, 2002)."[51] This study proposed that the stress of the vocation was the main factor in occupational burnout and showed that clergy are not only more obese but also more depressed. "The clergy depression prevalence was 8.7%, significantly higher than the 5.5% rate of the national sample."[52]

Longevity in ministry puts you more at risk. The same study tells us, "Longer time in ministry was related to more depression and anxiety. With a mean of 17 years in ministry, our sample of clergy is

---

50 Proeschold-Bell & LeGrand, 2010
http://divinity.duke.edu/sites/divinity.duke.edu/files/documents/chi/An%20Overview%20of%20the%20History%20and%20Current%20Status%20of%20Clergy%20Health_formatted.pdf

51
http://divinity.duke.edu/sites/divinity.duke.edu/files/documents/chi/An%20Overview%20of%20the%20History%20and%20Current%20Status%20of%20Clergy%20Health_formatted.pdf

52. Proeschold-Bell, R.J., Miles, A., Toth, M. Adams, C, Smith, B., & Toole, D. (2013). Using effort-reward imbalance theory to understand high rates of depression and anxiety among clergy. Journal of Primary Prevention, 34(6), 439-453. DOI: 10.1007/s10935-013-0321-4.

experienced, and has persisted in ministry; possibly this relation to more depression and anxiety can be explained by prolonged exposure to the stressful conditions mentioned above."[53]

The statistics show that clergy are at high risk because the role within our culture has become more complex requiring such a high number of competencies. Clergy are not the only caregivers to experience burnout. Doctors, ambulance drivers, counsellors, teachers, and indeed any who are in the caregiving area have potential for burnout. Other professions including police, military, and business leaders could be added to this group.

My psychiatrist kept asking me after I had partially resumed work, *"What was it that made me work so hard that I would become depleted?"* My first response was, "It's what we do; we work hard. It's the protestant work ethic, the pioneer spirit and all that. We make a way, put in the hard yards." It took me a long time to recognize that that wasn't how God wants me to live.

So how can organizations and leaders help their employees live a life God wants for them? This can be achieved in part by providing opportunities such as engaging mentors or spiritual directors; holding

---

[53]. http://divinity.duke.edu/sites/divinity.duke.edu/files/documents/chi/Clergy%20Depression%20%26%20Anxiety%20Effort-Reward%20Imbalance_formatted%20for%20web.pdf

retreats where workers can reflect on and reaffirm their calling; cultivating secure attachment relationships with their team and with God; and working through situations to determine the best coping strategies.

Congregations play a vital role in promoting the well-being of pastors. "Interestingly, clergy who experienced support from their congregations and anticipated that they would be supported if there were a future need, reported greater ministerial satisfaction and sense of personal accomplishment in ministry, but no less negative effect. Instead, it was the presence of demands from the congregation that was negatively affected. These findings suggest that to bolster positive affect optimally, congregations need to show support of their pastors to their pastors." [54]

Senior Leadership in a Church

It takes high performance people to lead a growing business or church. And high-performance people are those who are prone to burnout.

---

54. Duke Divinity School study http://divinity.duke.edu/initiatives/clergy-health-initiative/learning/

http://divinity.duke.edu/sites/divinity.duke.edu/files/documents/chi/2014%20Summary%20Report%20-%20CHI%20Statewide%20Survey%20of%20United%20Methodist%20Clergy%20in%20North%20Carolina%20-%20web.pdf

The senior leadership of a church is unique. A senior pastor feels the pressures that any high-level professional feels, emotionally and physically, while additionally carrying the spiritual weight.

I am passionate about Boards caring for their senior ministers as I have a deep desire to see churches be in good health and so fulfil the mission of Christ. However, often a Board will wrongly view the senior minister's engagement with the church and its vision as an indicator for how he is doing personally. My high engagement with the C3 movement and high buy-in to our church was clearly evident through the hours and resources I poured in. Yet all this masked what was happening to me internally. The load was not wise or sustainable. I wrongly thought that I was the one who should make up any deficit and carry any extra work and, thereby, hid my poor health. The level of responsibility I was carrying was too great.

During sessions with my psychiatrist, I unpacked many of the experiences that had seeded mistrust in the teams I worked with and the times I experienced broken trust. Over twenty years ago, close friends betrayed me, publicly and privately vilified me, rejected me so strongly that I could no longer minister at the church that had ordained me. When our C3 church started, two accountants on the team accused me of financial misconduct—this was proved unfounded by our public auditor. People who left the church mostly did so with blame and intense criticism.

What I didn't see was that these kinds of experiences made me close up for a long time. I was protective in what I let others know about myself and my experience. I realise now that I did not trust my Board with what was going on in me. In his book, *The Five Dysfunctions of a Team*, Patrick Lencioni says: "Trust is the foundation of real teamwork. And so, the first dysfunction is a failure on the part of team members to understand and open up to one another."[55] I have learnt that I can trust my Board, and I am endeavouring to be much more transparent.

My Psychologist really pushed me on my purpose and what I really want to accomplish: I needed to find my correct assignment. I knew that I wouldn't continue doing what I was before burnout. It was within that context that I rediscovered this scripture, Philippians 3:10-11: "I want to know Christ and experience the mighty power that raised him from the dead. I want to suffer with him, sharing in his death, so that one way or another I will experience the resurrection from the dead!" This scripture takes the pressure out of my

---

55 Lencioni, Patrick M.. *The Five Dysfunctions of a Team*, Enhanced Edition: A Leadership Fable (J-B Lencioni Series) (p. 43). Wiley. Kindle Edition.

performance as a minister and allows me to focus on my relationships. It reminds me that it's not about the numbers or financial gain; it is about the quality of connection.

What does well-being look like?

Without healthy examples, how do we know when we are not acting healthily? Or when our co-workers or employees or friends are silently asking for help? The expression of well-being can vary from person to person, and there is still much to discover about what it means to "be well". Once again, we look to Matt Bloom and Chris Adams in their article, *"Flourishing in Ministry: Well-being at Work in Helping Professions"*[56], as they take a deeper look into what allows most people to flourish. They found four elements that are key to living a happy and healthy life:

> *(1) an overarching system of beliefs, values and virtues that provides structure and guidance to life (meaning system)*
> *(2) a sense of contributing toward important purposes or goals in life (purpose in life)*
> *(3) an experience of being positively connected to others in mutually caring relationships (positive connectedness), and*

---

56 Adams & Bloom, Journal of Psychology and Christianity 2017, Vol. 36, No. 3, 254-259

(4) a positive self-concept (identity) and a sense of being one's true self, as well as striving to grow and improve as a person and achieving higher standards of virtue and excellence in one's life (authenticity & personal virtue)[57]

---

[57] Baumeister, 1991; Dutton, Roberts, & Bednar, 2010; Harter, 2002; Waterman & Schwartz, 2013

Reflection Questions for Chapter Five

1) How can I build self-awareness?
2) Who might be a potential mentor for me?
3) Who have my mentors been in the past?
4) What are my responsibilities at work regarding the well-being of others around me?
5) How can I take steps to protect my employees or co-workers from burnout?

CHAPTER SIX

Life After Burnout

Same but Different

I'm often asked, *"How are you doing now?"* The best answer I can give is that I'm the same but different. The whole process of burnout has changed me. This experience has burned away some of the rubbish and reshaped me. It has helped me begin to see what lay beneath the rubbish others and I placed on me. I know who I am, that first and foremost I am a child God. And that this is a gift not earned but accepted. So, I love to say, "I'm the same but different."

I discovered that the holes in my emotional tank affected my perceptions of myself—I spent years with a shallow sense of self-worth—and now I'm in the process of changing these perceptions. This makes me more relaxed both emotionally and physically. I am more assertive, this flowing out of deeper inner confidence. I'm learning to see things from God's perspective. I am a child of God, loved by Him. I know my purpose. I want to know Christ.[58] God values me, and the more I know of Him, the more I feel I can value myself how He values us all.

Some of my closest friends say to me, "I like the new you." They have noticed the change in me. However, I feel I'm not entirely new; part of my reflection here is that I *rediscovered* who I was. Things like the pressures and pain—they hurt yet focused me on my purpose. After burnout, I was able to connect to this again.

My emotions have come closer to the surface. Our cat passed away soon after I returned to work. Cookie was seventeen, and we'd had her since she was a kitten. We'd had cats for twenty years before her, and I have been very fond of all of them. But when Cookie died, my tears surprised me; deep groans poured from my soul at the loss of my faithful friend. The healing of emotions and soul that occurred through the journey of burnout and beyond helped me to grieve when I needed it.

Marvellous Mondays

These days, I begin my week with a Marvellous Monday. I have found

---

58. Philippians 3:10-11 New Living Translation (NLT) I want to know Christ and experience the mighty power that raised him from the dead. I want to suffer with him, sharing in his death, 11 so that one way or another I will experience the resurrection from the dead!

it incredibly helpful to calm my inner thoughts and refocus on what is important as I look towards the week ahead.

I start the day with breathing—some slow, deliberate inhales and exhales. (I make this my habit every day, not just Mondays.) I have a regular place where I sit. Sometimes, my cat curls on my lap. I read some verses from the Bible. I have shared that I like to use a Biblical "soundtrack"; a selection of key verses that speak to me about who I am and who God wants me to be. After I read my verses, I meditate on their meaning. I let myself be still and breathe.

I follow my meditation by asking myself some questions, really just checking in with myself. Here are the questions I come back to each week:

Reflecting

To reflect on the past week:

- What worked and what didn't?
- Where did I see the work of the Holy Spirit this week?
- Did the Lord nudge me in any way?
- In what ways could I change my actions to allow myself more replenishment and peace? (with the reminder to myself that I

am only responsible for what I can do, not for how others respond)

To reflect on my emotional well-being

- Check my gauges

Refocusing

To refocus on my core responsibilities:

- Current Projects
- Coaching (Leadership development)
- Connecting (Both in work and in my personal life)
- Celebrating (All the good things that God has given me)

Overview of what is coming up?

- What does this next week ask of me?
- When I feel emotionally strong, are there tough conversations or actions I need to plan for?
- Where can I schedule time to refill my tank?

Replenishing

- including an hour walk on the beach
- Adjust replenishing activities as needed

For more reading on the subject of creating a reflective routine, check out *"Two Things That Develop Self-reflection"* on the Verve Lead Blog.

The Gift of Burnout

I now consider burnout to be a gift. It has taken a couple of years to be able to see this. One of the questions people often ask is, "Have you recovered from burnout?" What people really want to know is, "Am I working? Am I stable? Is my life back to normal?" The short answer is yes, though I do many of the same things differently.

I have not returned to the same place I was before burnout. You cannot go back, but you can go on. Some might say I am weaker. My stamina is lower, and I need more time for replenishment. I realise there is much I don't know or see. Yet, in other ways, I am stronger, more aware. I have a greater understanding of myself, my God and the people around me. I have grown in self-confidence so that now I take criticisms far less personally. When someone is not doing well, I have eyes to see them and a quiet soul to help them through the storm. I am more settled and content with life, far less anxious and I am no longer striving to be what I am not. I am happy with my accomplishments that, at the end of the day, I can say with a smile, "I did well today." I feel content with the wonderful connections I am privileged to have been given.

These days, my tank has an overflow—I find I have something to give. My role is not to *do* primarily but to help others be their best. I have taken on more of a mentoring and coaching role in my work. I focus on making disciples who can engage in ministry and the world instead of simply being their minister. I feel my role has become almost paternal: like a parent's, my part is to teach, model and give more and more responsibility so that my people grow to be great people, parents and professionals. I am content and fulfilled in my new role.

It has been a challenging journey, going through the dark valley of burnout. I would never wish to inflict the pain of this on anyone. However, as I reflect on this now, I have to say, "Thank you for the gift of burnout."

I don't reply that I am back from burnout, but I've gone beyond.

A bigger plan than me

I hope that it will significantly benefit you as you read this story. It can be hard to see your purpose, to understand how you can make a difference in your life and others when going through this difficult time. The pain may be intense even while you experience numbness. It is hard to see anything beyond you, let alone to think how this fits in with others' journey other than seeing the pain you also are causing in them. I can see that the stress, anxiety and depression had real causes. I didn't just randomly break, but a combination of my choices and others' responses and actions had seriously affected me. I felt out of control, sliding downwards, heading into a dark pit with deep walls, so slippery that I couldn't find a foothold to climb out. It was only through reflection, rest and the support of my friends and family that I could recover. These were my footholds. It took a great deal of candour and transparency from myself and those around me to reconcile my past and present self. I am so grateful.

I love the thought that through our own difficulties, we can actually become something beneficial to other people. 2 Corinthians 1:3-5 says just this in The Message Version, entitled *The Rescue*:

> *"All praise to the God and Father of our Master, Jesus the Messiah! Father of all mercy! God of all healing counsel! He comes alongside us when we go through hard times, and before you know it, he brings us alongside someone else who is going through hard times so that we can be there for that person just as God was there for us. We have plenty of hard times that come from following the Messiah, but no more so than the good times of his healing comfort—we get a full measure of that, too."* [59]

Martin Luther is a great example of this passage. In 1527, his town was

---

[59] 2 Corinthians 1:3-5 The Message (MSG)

struck with the Bubonic Plague; and pandemics are a devastating occurrence in any age! Martin Luther couldn't preach publicly as it would have been dangerous to himself and his congregation. However, this led him to procure a printing press (still very new technology at the time) which enabled the distribution of his thoughts and ideas in ways he had not been able to do with preaching in a church. There is no denying that this catastrophic pandemic was tragic, but good came from it also. Our life's struggles allow us to make new connections, to become more creative, inventive, empathetic and appreciative.

It's clear to me that through all this, there is a much bigger purpose, a larger hand, at work. When we'd been meeting for about twelve months, my psychologist said he had a story to tell me. He asked, "Do you know how I got to be a psychologist?" I had no idea. He said, "Don, your ministry has had much more effect than you realise. More people's lives have been influenced for the better than you know." He told me about a man he had known, Chris, who happened to be on my pastoral team. "Well, several years ago, he was listening to my aspirations and said to me, 'Greg, go see your dream become reality. Make it happen, go do that course of study, go to university and become the person you see in your dream.' So, I'm here today as a psychologist to help you back to health because one of your team members spoke to me. You've sown seeds, and those seeds have borne fruit. That fruit has sown seeds that now you receive the benefit of."

I was speechless, so impacted by the story. I was just at a point in my recovery where I was beginning to see a renewed purpose for my life. What I had spent my life, energy and actions on was not wasted: it was actually of great significance. I've already mentioned how I rediscovered delight in helping people to know God, and my psychologist helped me discover that I love helping people find a purpose for their lives.

You can imagine the impact of this. I was overwhelmed with a feeling that everything was okay—even the bad stuff. God was there looking out for me, and more than that, He was working all things together for good. He set up Chris to speak to Greg, so Greg could be there to talk to me. Amazing! Every time I think of this or tell this story, I feel safe.

Greg has told this story publicly and thanked Chris for his quiet behind-the-scenes encouragement that calls the best out of people.

My purpose in writing *Burnout and Beyond* is to help you. You may find yourself in burnout, but you will go beyond. Someone is looking out for you—and not just someone, but the One, the Father who loves you. May these words give you hope, courage and peace.

Reflection Questions for Chapter Six

1) How has the journey through burnout changed me?
2) In what way have I changed my life to better care for my well-being?
3) Who has helped me? How can I thank them?
4) Who might I have hurt during my burnout? How can I make reparations?
5) How can I use my experience to help others?

THANK YOU

Thank You Letters

Physiotherapists:

Thank you, for being part of God's healing and blessing for me. When I began the time off, I knew that the Lord is my Shepherd, and I would not want. But I had no idea of how that would happen/work.

You both, your professional ability, who you are, and the grace of God flowing through you have helped to renew my strength. So, my declaration is:

> *"He renews my strength. He guides me along the right paths, bringing honour to his name." Ps 23:3*

As I am bringing honour to His name in the days to come, smile, knowing that you have been part of this.

Love and Blessings,

Ps Dr Don Easton

Psychologist: Greg Gardiner

Thank you, for being part of God's healing and blessing for me.

Thank you, for helping me to rest, to hear the permission of heaven, "He lets me rest." Ps 23:2 NLT

Thank you for helping me breathe, enjoy the green meadows and peaceful streams.

Thank you for helping me see who I truly am, that my head is anointed, my cup is overflowing, I'm pursued by goodness and unfailing love and that I live in the house of the Lord forever.

Greg, you have been an instrument of heaven; for rest, restoring, and refuelling. Thank you.

Love and Blessings,
Ps Dr Don Easton

Letter of Apology

To any affected by my sickness,

Firstly, thank you for your part in building C3 Church Robina.

When I think of the journey we shared, a smile comes on my face, and my heart feels full of deep affection. Your sacrifice and ministry in our church have contributed to the wonderful community of faith it is today.

Secondly, I write to give a personal apology. Recently, I have come to see some of the pain I caused you.

In a few years before 2014, I became increasingly unwell. I avoided any conflict and withdrew. My emotional depletion caused many to become dry and depleted. I recognise I failed you, and I am sorry that my best at that time was not enough for you.

Sorry for any grief or pain that I caused.

I write this as I desire to see you thrive in your relationship with God and flourish in all your connections.

May inner strength be yours and His power work mightily through you. This is my prayer for you:

Ephesians 3:16-21

> *16 I pray that from his glorious, unlimited resources, he will empower you with inner strength through his Spirit. 17 Then Christ will make his home in your hearts as you trust in him. Your roots will grow down into God's love and keep you strong. 18 And may you have the power to understand, as all*

God's people should, how wide, how long, how high, and how deep his love is. 19 May you experience the love of Christ, though it is too great to understand fully. Then you will be made complete with all the fullness of life and power that comes from God.

20 Now all glory to God, who is able, through his mighty power at work within us, to accomplish infinitely more than we might ask or think. 21 Glory to him in the church and in Christ Jesus through all generations forever and ever! Amen.

Love and Blessings,

Don

REFERENCES

Proeschold-Bell, Rae Jean, et al. "Using Effort-Reward Imbalance Theory to Understand High Rates of Depression and Anxiety among Clergy." *Https://Divinity.duke.edu*, 22 Aug. 2013, https://divinity.duke.edu/sites/divinity.duke.edu/files/documents/chi/Clergy%20Depression%20%26%20Anxiety%20Effort-Reward%20Imbalance_formatted%20for%20web.pdf.

Adams, Chris, and Matt Bloom. "Flourishing in Ministry: Wellbeing at Work in Helping Professions." *Journal of Psychology and Christianity*, vol. 36, 2017, pp. 254–258., https://doi.org/https://www.crcna.org/sites/default/files/adams_bloom_jpc_fall_2017_article.pdf.

Bloom, Matt. *A Burden Too Heavy? Research Insights from the Flourishing in Ministry Project*. University of Notre Dame, 2017.

Bradberry, Travis, and Jean Greaves. *Emotional Intelligence 2.0*. TalentSmart, 2009.

"Burn-out an 'Occupational Phenomenon': International Classification of Diseases." *World Health Organization*, World Health Organization, 28 May 2019, https://www.who.int/news/item/28-05-2019-burn-out-an-occupational-phenomenon-international-classification-of-diseases.

Chris, Adams, and Bloom Matt. "Flourishing in Ministry: Wellbeing at Work in Helping Professions." *Journal of Psychology and Christianity*, vol. 36, 2017, pp. 254–259.

"Community Driver Reviver." *NSW*, 12 Nov. 2021, http://roadsafety.transport.nsw.gov.au/stayingsafe/fatigue/driverreviver/index.html.

Covey, Stephen R. *Wisdom and Teachings of Stephen R. Covey*. Simon & Schuster Ltd, 2012.

George, Carl F. *How to Break Growth Barriers: Revise Your Role, Release Your People, and Capture Overlooked ... Opportunities for Your Church*. Baker Book House, 2017.

Hart, Archibald D. *The Hidden Link between Adrenalin & Stress: The*

Exciting New Breakthrough That Helps You Overcome Stress Damage. Kindle Edition ed., Thomas Nelson, 1995.

Hart, Archibald D., and Sharon Morris May. *Safe Haven Marriage: A Marriage You Can Come Home To*. W Pub. Group, 2003.

Hybels, Bill. *Courageous Leadership*. Zondervan, 2012.

"Job Description for Church Staff: Tony Cooke Ministries." *Tony Cooke Ministries | Articles for Church Leaders | Ministry & Leadership Resources*, 8 Dec. 2020, http://www.tonycooke.org/stories-and-illustrations/job_description/.

Lencioni, Patrick M. *The Five Dysfunctions of a Team: A Leadership Fable*. Enhanced Edition ed., John Wiley & Sons, 2007.

Lewis, Rick. "Page 183." *Mentoring Matters*, Monarch Books, Grand Rapids, MI, 2009.

"List of Fatal Snake Bites in Australia." *Wikipedia*, Wikimedia Foundation, 9 Oct. 2021, https://en.wikipedia.org/wiki/List_of_fatal_snake_bites_in_Australia.

Moore, Gordon. *Going to the Next Level*. Ark House Press, 2015.

Proeschold-Bell, Rae Jean. "An Overview of the History and Current Status of Clergy Health." *Https://Divinity.duke.edu*, Duke Global Health Institute, https://divinity.duke.edu/sites/divinity.duke.edu/files/documents/chi/An%20Overview%20of%20the%20History%20and%20Current%20Status%20of%20Clergy%20Health_formatted.pdf.

Proeschold-Bell, Rae, et al. "The Glory of God Is a Human Being Fully Alive: Predictors of Positive versus Negative Mental Health among Clergy." *Journal for the Scientific Study of Religion*, vol. 54, no. 4, 2015, pp. 702–721., https://doi.org/10.1111/jssr.12234.

"Protestant Ethic." *Encyclopædia Britannica*, Encyclopædia Britannica, Inc., 20 July 1998, https://www.britannica.com/topic/Protestant-ethic.

"Related Psychological Health and Safety: A Systematic Approach to Meeting Your Duties." *safeworkaustralia.gov.au/Topic/Mental-Health*, 1 Jan. 2019, https://www.safeworkaustralia.gov.au/doc/work-related-psychological-health-and-safety-systematic-approach-meeting-your-duties.

Riley, Philip, and Sioau-Mai See. "The Australian Principal Occupational Health, Safety and Wellbeing Survey." *Health and Wellbeing.org*, Institute for Positive Psychology and Education Australian Catholic University, Feb. 2020, https://www.healthandwellbeing.org/reports/AU/2019%20ACU%20Australian%20Principals%20Report.pdf.

The Rolling Stones. "(I Can't Get No) Satisfaction." *On Air*, 1965.

Seppälä, Emma, and Julia Moeller. "1 In 5 Employees Is Highly Engaged and at Risk of Burnout." *Harvard Business Review*, 16 May 2018, https://hbr.org/2018/02/1-in-5-highly-engaged-employees-is-at-risk-of-burnout.

Siegel, Dr Dan. "The Developing Mind: How Relationships and the Brain Interact to Shape Who We Are." Second Edition. *Dr Dan Siegel*, 18 Apr. 2021, https://drdansiegel.com/.

Valcour, Monique. "4 Steps to Beating Burnout." *Harvard Business Review*, 27 Aug. 2021, https://hbr.org/2016/11/beating-burnout.

Vasagar, Jeevan. "Out of Hours Working Banned by German Labour Ministry." *The Telegraph*, Telegraph Media Group, 30 Aug. 2013, http://www.telegraph.co.uk/news/worldnews/europe/germany/10276815/Out-of-hours-working-banned-by-German-labour-ministry.html.

ABOUT DON

Dr Don Easton has dedicated much time to the exploration and analysis of burnout in Christian leaders, after enduring burnout firsthand in 2014. His own experience with burnout and recovery led to a deep passion to increase the buoyancy and well-being of Christian leaders, making these leaders and their communities stronger, healthier and more resilient. With forty-five years of ministry and formal Doctoral education at Fuller Theological Seminary, Don is distinctively positioned to recognize the complexities and pressures of modern Christian leaders.

Don is currently the Senior Minister for C3 Church Robina, a well-being mentor, a professional supervisor, consultant and author. Early during the Covid-19 pandemic, he founded the charity Vervelead.com to promote mentoring, the development of mentors and well-being procedures in organisations. Pastors, Principals, Politicians, and Business leaders value what he brings.

Don and Adrienne married in 1979 and have three married children and seven grandchildren.

Don completed a Graduate Certificate of Professional Supervision in 2021 and is an associate of Australian Association of Supervision.

Don is a member of the Australian Christian Mentoring Network.

www.ingramcontent.com/pod-product-compliance
Lightning Source LLC
Chambersburg PA
CBHW071710020426
42333CB00017B/2201